Dr. Lacouture's
Skin Care
Guide

for

People Living
With Cancer

Mario E. Lacouture, MD

*Forewords by Cornelia Dean
and Steven T. Rosen, MD, FACP*

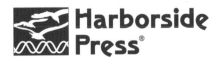

**Harborside
Press®**

Dr. Lacouture's Skin Care Guide for People Living With Cancer

by Mario E. Lacouture, MD

Publisher
Harborside Press, LLC
37 Main Street
Cold Spring Harbor, NY 11724
www.HarborsidePress.com

Library of Congress Control Number: 2012940001

Trademarks
All terms mentioned in this book that are known to be trademarks or service marks have been appropriately capitalized. Harborside Press cannot attest to the accuracy of this information. Use of a term in the book should not be regarded as affecting the validity of any trademark or service mark.

Disclaimer
The information and reference materials contained herein are for general informational purposes and not intended to take the place of professional medical care. Moreover, the information in this volume is not intended to dictate what constitutes reasonable, appropriate, or best care for any given health issue, but rather, should be considered as a basis for discussion with one's own physician. This information should not be considered medical advice and is not intended to replace consultation with a qualified medical professional. Patients should not change or modify their disease management plan without consulting their treating physicians. The author and editors have made every effort to provide information that is accurate and complete as of the date of publication. However, given the rapid changes occurring in medical science, as well as the possibility of human error, this book may contain technical inaccuracies or other errors. The author, editors, and publishers will not be liable for any direct or indirect damages arising therefrom.

First printing: May 2012

Illustrated by DNA Illustrations and Michael Buckley
Layout artists: Sarah McGullam and Gail van Koot

ISBN: 978-0-615-45226-5

10   9   8   7   6   5   4   3   2   1

This book is printed in the United States of America on acid-free paper conforming to ANSI/NISO Z39.48-1992 standards for paper permanence.

To the memory of my father,
my greatest teacher and mentor

Contents

A Patient's Foreword

In September 2010, Dr. Mario Lacouture asked me to help teach some of his fellow dermatologists about the skin effects of cancer treatment—and how they could help their patients deal with them. In the seminar Dr. Lacouture conducted at Memorial Sloan-Kettering Cancer Center, the visiting doctors marveled at the cracked skin on my feet, my damaged toenails, rashes, dozens of lesions on my arms and legs, and two oozing skin infections.

"Wow," one of the doctors said after reviewing this catalogue of symptoms. "You really had everything, didn't you?"

That was an understatement. In the course of my treatment for breast cancer—which included chemotherapy, a double mastectomy, radiation therapy, and reconstruction—side effects to my skin posed one challenge after another. But Dr. Lacouture was able to deal with all of it. And now that my cancer treatment is over, I can tell you: **Even if you have the many side effects that I did, your doctor can ease your way through it, too.**

When I was diagnosed in 2009, I knew from a lifetime of experience that my delicate skin would be an issue. When I was 18, one doctor told me that my dry skin was the worst he had ever seen and wondered aloud, "How can you stand it?" Wool, wool blends, and even cashmere gave me a rash. My childhood summers were one burning, peeling sunburn after another. Everything from plants to metals irritated my skin.

So it was no surprise to me that my skin reacted as it did to cancer treatment. Luckily, my medical oncologist, Dr.

Larry Norton, referred me to Dr. Lacouture, who had just joined the staff at Sloan-Kettering from the Robert H. Lurie Comprehensive Cancer Center of Northwestern University, where he was the Director of the Cancer Skin Program.

What brought me to him initially were angry skin infections on my chest and left arm. It was not immediately obvious what was wrong with me. I was pale and weak but just thought that was because of my chemotherapy.

Before I left the clinic that day, Dr. Lacouture ordered some blood work. By the time I staggered into a cab and got across town to my apartment, my phone was ringing. It was my oncology nurse. Come back to the hospital, she told me. I was dangerously short of infection-fighting white blood cells. After a four-day hospital stay and IV antibiotics, I was healthy enough to be released.

By then, Dr. Lacouture had determined that the skin infections were a result of a condition called Sweet's syndrome. He prescribed antibiotics and topical corticosteroids, and the infections went away. But the skin infections meant I could not stick to my chemotherapy treatment plan. My oncologist had to come up with another idea.

Soon, though, squamous cell skin cancers started appearing all over my body—and quickly. I had had skin cancer before, many times in fact. But this outbreak was different. One day, I found at least 20 skin cancer lesions on my right shin alone. Once again, Dr. Lacouture explained this condition to me and prescribed medications. Eventually, the skin cancers faded.

Meanwhile, the skin on my hands and feet was cracking, and my toenails were separating from the nail beds. One day, while on a visit to another Sloan-Kettering doctor, I stopped in at Dr. Lacouture's office and asked him to look at the nail on my right big toe. Although it wasn't exactly separated, it wasn't really attached either. He was sympathetic. "Would you like me to take it off?" he asked. More than a year later, it has almost finished growing back.

My guess is that many people with cancer dismiss these symptoms as annoyances rather than real problems. That was definitely my view, and I was reluctant to bring them up during office visits. I did not want to come across as a patient who was easily annoyed and quick to complain. But my doctors and nurses set me straight on this. **Telling your clinician about a problem is not complaining. It is reporting.** Often, your report contains information that your doctors and nurses need to know.

Yes, plenty of cancer problems are worse than detaching toenails. But loose toenails are no fun, especially if your feet are already numb from chemotherapy-related neuropathy and you are coping with aching bones or other side effects of treatment. And, as Dr. Lacouture tells us in this book, there are ways to manage these side effects and make them go away. **If you can relieve your discomfort, you should.** It will improve your quality of life and enable you to complete your treatment.

This book guides patients (and their clinicians too) through this journey. It tells about the biology of skin and cancer and describes how cancer and its treatments—chemotherapy, radiation therapy, and surgery—can damage skin, hair, and nails.

It describes rashes, hives, pimples, redness, dryness, and itching. It describes hair loss, radiation burns, and scarring from surgery. The book covers discolored, brittle, and bleeding nails and nails that loosen and separate. It describes the skin conditions that often follow stem cell transplants.

Some of these conditions have little to do with your cancer itself. Some conditions, such as hair loss, affect your psyche more than anything else. But sometimes, as was the case with my skin infection, they are signs of something serious.

As Dr. Lacouture explains here, skin side effects can be signs that your treatment is working well. In fact, that's what my oncologist Dr. Norton told me about side effects in general. Think of it this way, he said: The bad news is your body is really sensitive to these treatments, and you are having all these side effects. The good news is your body is really sensitive to these treatments, and the cancer is gone.

Given the choice, I'll take side effects and no cancer over the reverse.

When Dr. Lacouture asked me to take part in the 2010 seminar, I was happy to oblige. Although I was a good example of what can happen to the skin as a result of cancer treatment, I was also a good example of how much can be done to reduce these side effects and make them easier to bear.

The doctors who looked at my cracked, oozing, and inflamed skin were seeing it in color photos displayed on a computer screen. I could tell them what had happened and describe what it felt like, but I spoke in the past tense. The damage to my skin had healed to the point that I could not say exactly where on my chest and arms those dreadful infections had been. **There were no lingering signs on my skin to tell me.**

When I look back on my treatment, the only emotion that comes to mind is gratitude for all the people who helped me through it. Dr. Lacouture was one of those people. Through his book, he will help many others.

Cornelia Dean
New York, NY
April 2012

A Physician's Foreword

The treatment of cancer has evolved dramatically over the past few decades, and many current therapies are much more effective than what was available years ago. As a result, the number of survivors has increased greatly. But one of the consequences of some modern treatments has been side effects that affect the skin, hair, or nails—both short- and long-term. Because these areas of the body are visible, such side effects can be very distressing. Cosmetic issues affect intimacy and quality of life. In some cases, symptoms of the skin or nails can cause pain and affect function, interfering with work or daily activities.

It is important for all patients and cancer survivors to be aware of the side effects of cancer therapies and how to minimize or treat them as needed. This is an area of dermatology that is still evolving, and many physicians are new to the scientific literature in the field. That is why my colleague, Dr. Mario Lacouture, an expert in this area, has written this book. He understands that, with the support of loved ones, patients are their own best advocates. Armed with the information in this book, people with cancer can work with their doctors to make the best possible choices in preventing and treating cancer-related side effects.

Steven T. Rosen, MD, FACP
Director, Robert H. Lurie
Comprehensive Cancer Center
Chicago, Illinois
April 2012

Author's Preface

During my dermatology residency training at the University of Chicago, I was asked to see a patient being treated for kidney cancer with an experimental medication that was causing a severe rash on the face and painful blisters on the hands and feet. After the oncologist left the exam room so I could conduct the examination, the patient exclaimed, "Doctor, please give me something for my rash and the pain on my hands and feet. If this doesn't improve, my oncologist will stop the chemotherapy. I want to be there for my daughter's wedding. I'll do anything, but please, help me stay on this medication."

This conversation is what it took for me to realize that despite the advances and immense contributions that had been made for decades by scientists and oncologists, and even more remarkable medical discoveries in the past few years, something had been overlooked, although it is the most visible human organ: the skin.

For obvious reasons, the skin, hair, and nails have not been topmost concerns in oncology—the most important goal is to treat and cure the cancer. But skin conditions in people living with cancer can affect their sense of self and their interactions with others, and these side effects can lead to costly treatments and affect overall health. Perhaps most critically, in many cases (up to half of all people receiving some of the newer medications), anticancer treatments need to be reduced or stopped because of skin conditions arising as a consequence of therapies. Taken together, these factors have led to the establishment of dermatologic care as a necessary component of cancer therapies.

When I decided to dedicate myself to participating in the care of people living with cancer, I never imagined the need for the information in this book and the impact that it would have on so many people and their families. What has made this so rewarding is that people always tell me about the effect that optimally maintaining their skin, hair, and nails has on their lives and their ability to receive treatment. People undergoing chemotherapy or radiation therapy who had rashes all over their body were now able to go to work; others with painful nails could cook for their family; and those with blisters on hands and feet were now capable of exercise, to name a few examples of the comments I've heard from patients.

But reducing or preventing dermatologic side effects does not end at the physical level. Many people tell me how the improvement in their skin has improved their quality of life, their interaction with others, their confidence, and most significantly, their ability to enjoy each and every day. Although participating in the care of the skin, hair, and nails in people living with cancer is but a part of the remarkable work that oncologists do, it is a significant one.

I am honored to be able to participate in the care of people living with cancer, alongside many esteemed and brilliant oncology and dermatology colleagues. My dedication and interest in this emerging field of medicine would not have been possible without amazing mentors: Keo Soltani, Christopher Shea, Lloyd Klickstein, George Hambrick, Allan Halpern, Amy Paller, and Steven Rosen. All of them are supportive, dedicated physicians who encouraged me to follow my passion where dermatology and oncology intersect. After attending many oncology meetings, I am flabbergasted at oncologists' devotion and constancy in seeking knowledge, so that they can make people's lives better and longer.

I would also like to acknowledge the contributions of Conor Lynch, Susan Reckling, Randi Londer Gould, David Horowitz, Jack Gentile, Anthony Cutrone, and the rest of the team at Harborside Press for all of their efforts in bringing this book to publication.

Most importantly, I feel privileged to be able to participate in the care of so many courageous people, who together with their families, share with me what is most valuable in their lives, and how improving their skin allows them to achieve that. I am wordless at their altruism, when they allow me to examine, photograph, or biopsy their skin so that we can have a better understanding, or when they contact me about what skin regimen worked for them, so that I can share that information with others who have similar conditions.

With best wishes during
this journey,

Mario E. Lacouture, MD
New York, NY
May 2012

About this Book

If you are a person living with cancer, you may experience changes in your skin, hair, or nails. These changes may be associated with cancer itself or as a result of cancer treatments. Some people may experience these side effects months—or even years—after their treatment for cancer is finished. This book has been written to help you understand and manage any of the potential changes to your skin, hair, or nails.

In this book, you will find practical advice on how to cope with these symptoms, which can range from mild and annoying to severe enough to affect your health and quality of life. In some cases, they are so serious that cancer treatments must be stopped, at least until the symptoms are brought under control. That's why it is so important to work with your healthcare team to prevent and manage these changes if they appear. There are many effective medications your doctor can prescribe, as well as over-the-counter products that you can use to prevent and treat many skin conditions in people living with cancer, steps that will improve your skin's health, your well-being, and even your outlook on life.

The information provided in these pages comes from over a decade of caring for people living with cancer. During this time, I carefully recorded the clinical presentation, treatment, and outcome of dozens of different skin, hair, and nail conditions in both patients and long-term survivors. I have also read hundreds of articles from medical journals in the oncology, dermatology, and supportive care literature. In many cases, the conditions that I would need to treat were completely new—they had never been described before in any medical article or textbook. In these cases, I would extrapolate from information on disorders that had a similar appearance in people who were not living with cancer. Other times, I was the beneficiary of my patients' courage and altruism: they would share the names of effective creams or products, or describe the successful methods they were using to alleviate their condition, so that I could pass on this knowledge to other people living with cancer.

In the chapters that follow, I will discuss the most common skin, hair, and nail side effects from cancer treatment. You'll learn the best ways to care for these conditions before, during, and after your treatment. Maybe this is the most important lesson to be learned from this book: **there are many effective ways to prevent and manage these side effects so that they do not disrupt your quality of life or interfere with your cancer treatment.**

In each chapter, I've combined the latest medical research with my own experience in treating people. The book contains numerous tables, sidebars, and illustrations that help you get the knowledge you need in a manner that's comfortable for you. Each chapter has helpful (and sometimes quirky) information in sidebars tagged "Did You Know?" and a box summarizing the key points at the end of the chapter labeled "Things to Remember." There's a glossary of medical terms on page 259, a list of anti-cancer medications with their generic and brand names on page 247, and references for more information on page 271. The information contained in this book is intended for discussions with your doctor or nurse. These healthcare professionals are important allies when it comes to treating your symptoms.

Taken as a whole, the facts gathered in this book are the result of caring for people living with cancer. I feel privileged to have participated in the care of many wonderful individuals and their families throughout the years, people who have shown me unremitting humanity in the face of serious challenges to their health. I hope this book will help you and your loved ones learn what to expect during your cancer journey, and how you can best care for your skin, hair, and nails before, during, and after treatment, so that you can make the most out of every day.

Mario E. Lacouture, MD
New York, NY
May 2012

CHAPTER 1

Understanding Your Skin

There are many reasons why skin, hair, and nail conditions are so frequent in people living with cancer. First, any chemotherapy that is administered either orally or through a vein will make its way into the skin, affecting the way it works. Second, because these changes appear in visible areas of the body, people are more likely to notice them and become concerned. Third, the skin and cancer, unfortunately, share some similarities: they are abundantly nourished by blood and are composed of rapidly growing cells, all of which make them susceptible to any of the three primary tools used against cancer: chemotherapy, radiation, and surgery.

If that were not enough, nearly one out of two people will have some sort of skin disease before starting treatment. These conditions are usually mild and include dry skin, itching, or skin infections—all of which may become aggravated during treatment.

This introductory chapter explains the basics on:
- the biology of skin and its functions
- cancer cells and their growth
- how cancer and its treatment can affect the skin, hair, and nails.

The Skin and Its Functions

The skin is the body's largest organ, accounting for 15 percent of our weight; it is perhaps one of the most diverse organs as well—thickest on the soles of the feet

DID YOU KNOW?

The entire surface of the skin measures about 20 square feet, and all of the body's skin weighs between seven and nine pounds.

and palms of the hands and thinnest on the eyelids. The skin forms our hair and nails, and it changes continually, completely renewing itself about once a month.

Skin can reflect our mood and physical well-being; it contributes to our sense of self and the way the world sees us. The skin also has many responsibilities: it helps protect us from heat, cold, chemicals, infectious bacteria, yeast, viruses, and damaging rays from the sun. It enables our sense of touch, helps regulate our body temperature, and controls the loss of fluids.

The skin is made up of three different layers, stacked on top of each another:

Epidermis This thin outermost layer is about as thick as a business card. It contains layers of cells that grow and slough off every month. This process ensures that our epidermis remains relatively new throughout our lives. One protein made within the cells of the epidermis is called keratin. It is the strongest protein in the skin and acts like a shield. Not only does keratin protect the skin from chemicals and infections, it also bundles together to form hair and nails, giving them their strength. Keratin-forming cells make up the bulk of the epidermis. Other types of cells include melanocytes (pigment-forming cells) and dendritic cells. Melanocytes produce melanin, which gives skin its color. Dendritic cells are part of the immune system; they capture bacteria and viruses before they can cause disease.

Dermis This middle layer of skin is thicker than the epidermis, measuring about 1/8 of an inch (or a stack of two business cards). In the dermis, substances such as elastin and collagen, which lend structure and support to the skin, are produced. Elastin makes it possible for skin to be flexible, and collagen gives skin its strength (75 percent of the dermis is made up of collagen). Hair follicles (or roots), as well as a network of oil and sweat glands, are found in the dermis. The dermis also contains nerves for touch and temperature sensing, as well as blood vessels, which provide nutrition to the skin.

Hypodermis The deepest part of the skin, this layer is made up mostly of fat. The hypodermis helps insulate the body, carry blood vessels, and protect internal organs.

Cancer Cells and Their Growth

Healthy cells in the body (including those in the skin) grow and divide in a controlled way. They line up in an orderly fashion, working together to help each other function correctly as an organ. When it's time to stop growing, cells receive a signal that they have reached their "limit." Cells are also programmed either to repair themselves or die if the skin is injured or damaged.

But cancer cells do not obey these rules. They grow uncontrollably, ignoring signals that tell them when it is time to stop. In addition, they repeatedly produce new cells with genetic mutations (errors in the body's DNA code, which programs cell func-

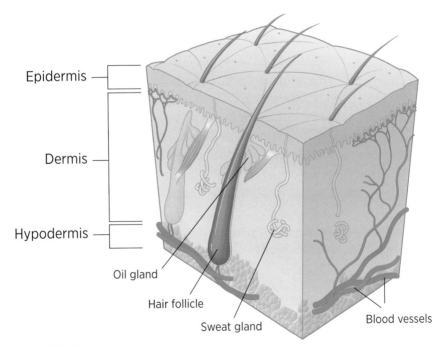

Epidermis

Dermis

Hypodermis

Oil gland

Hair follicle

Sweat gland

Blood vessels

A CLOSER LOOK AT THE SKIN
The skin is made up of three different layers: the epidermis, dermis, and hypodermis. Hair follicles, oil and sweat glands, and blood vessels are all important parts of the skin.

tions). When cancer cells reproduce, they pass along their mutations to their offspring, or "daughter" cells, which sometimes even take on new errors. Cancer cells also move to different parts of the body and take the place of healthy cells. In order to stay alive, they attract their own nourishing blood vessels. The challenge in treating cancer lies in the fact that every person's cancer is unique, with its own pattern of growth and response to treatment.

There are various types of cancers that can occur in the body, with nearly as many causes. Cancer often arises as a result of a complex interaction among genes, the environment, and lifestyle choices. For example, exposure to certain industrial pollutants, pesticides, and viral infections can lead to cancer. Personal choices such as smoking, diet, and sun exposure play a role in the development of other cancers. In fact, up to one third of cancers could be prevented if people ate a healthful diet, maintained an ideal weight, avoided excessive sun exposure, and did not smoke.

Scientists have learned a great deal about cancers that run in families, especially breast, ovarian, colorectal, kidney, nerve, blood, some types of eye, and skin cancers, including melanoma. Inherited mutations—passed from parents to children, putting affected family members at a higher cancer risk—are a small percentage (less than one in ten) of all cancers.

Q Because I've never had any problems with my skin, hair, or nails, I was surprised when I developed side effects from my cancer treatment. Are these types of problems to be expected?

A Yes, but for the most part, they can be managed. A survey of cancer survivors showed that 67 percent did not expect skin problems to occur prior to treatment. But once they finished their treatment, skin irritation and dry skin were reported as the most common side effects. Since most anti-cancer treatments work by destroying rapidly growing cancer cells, healthy skin cells will also be affected.

Even before my cancer was diagnosed, I noticed changes in my skin, hair, and nails. How do I know whether these changes were related to the cancer? And will treating my cancer improve these problems?

Many conditions such as dry and itchy skin, brittle nails, and hair loss naturally occur with age. And because up to 80 percent of cancers are diagnosed in people over the age of 50, it's difficult to know whether aging or the cancer is responsible. In one out of 100 people, changes in the skin are linked to cancer, and they are known as paraneoplastic (from the Greek words *para*, which means alongside, and *neoplasia*, which means new growth). Paraneoplastic skin conditions will usually improve when the underlying cancer is treated.

Cancers that arise in the lungs, head and neck, colon and rectum, breasts, or ovaries may spread (metastasize) to the skin but are not considered to be skin cancers. If these cancers spread to the skin, they are treated in the same way as they were before. In some cases, surgery or radiation therapy can be used to treat cancers that have spread to the skin.

Regarding skin cancers, the two most common types are basal and squamous cell carcinomas. They occur as a result of exposure to the sun or radiation treatments. More than 2 million people are diagnosed with skin cancers every year in the United States. Fortunately, basal and squamous cell cancers rarely spread or become life-threatening.

Melanoma is a much more serious form of skin cancer. It affects about 75,000 people a year in the United States and can be life-threatening. Melanoma may begin with moles that change; if left untreated, melanoma can spread to other organs. Diagnosing melanoma early is vitally important, so changes in moles must be monitored carefully. Many people living with cancer will have a heightened risk of developing skin cancer. This may occur as a result of anti-cancer treatments or the cancer itself affecting the immune system, which helps fight off skin cancers.

DID YOU KNOW?

As we grow older, the body makes less elastin and collagen, which is the reason why the skin starts to wrinkle and sag. This process can sometimes be more noticeable after receiving chemotherapy.

Skin Conditions Associated With Cancer

These conditions can occur in people with a family history of diseases that heighten the risk of cancer and specific skin changes (the so-called inherited cancer syndromes) or with paraneoplastic syndromes (in which the cancer itself affects the skin), both of which are rare disorders. Talk to your doctor about appropriate cancer tests based on your health and family history, and consult with a dermatologist about any skin changes.

If you have...	It may be associated with...
Spots that are brown to black	Breast, ovarian, testicular, uterine, cervical, gastrointestinal cancers, lymphomas, leukemias
Hot flashes	Neuroendocrine cancers
Dark, velvety, or thick skin in creases	Stomach, lung, cervical, breast cancers
Excessive hair growth	Stomach, urinary, colorectal cancers, leukemias
Thick skin on the palms	Lung, stomach, head and neck, colorectal cancers
Itching	Lymphomas
Round red spots	Lung, esophageal, breast cancers
Blisters	Lymphomas, leukemias, bone cancers
Purple eyelid discoloration, redness on the cuticles or back	Ovarian, breast, uterine, lung, stomach, colorectal, pancreatic cancers
Yellow bumps on the face	Genitourinary, colorectal, breast, kidney, endometrial, thyroid cancers, leukemias
Skin-colored bumps/cysts	Colorectal, kidney cancers
Dark spots on the lips	Gastrointestinal cancers

How Cancer and Its Treatment Can Affect the Skin, Hair, and Nails: An Overview

Changes in the skin may be an early warning sign that cancer is present in other parts of the body. For example, people with inherited cancer syndromes of the stomach, gallbladder, or pancreas may have a long-standing history of brown to black spots on the lips or

DOs AND DON'Ts WHEN STARTING TREATMENT

DO

- Ask your doctor or nurse if the medicine you will be receiving is associated with dermatologic (skin, hair, and nail) side effects.
- Make a list of side effects that should prompt a call to your doctor or a trip to the hospital.
- Take your medicines as instructed.
- Keep a diary of when you develop side effects.
- Inform your oncologist and any of your other doctors of any medicines, vitamins, or supplements you are taking.

DON'T

- Skip doses or take more doses than prescribed.
- Start other medications, vitamins, or supplements during treatment unless you first discuss it with your oncologist.
- Stop taking preventive anti-allergy medications (antihistamines, corticosteroids) that are prescribed by your doctor just because you have not experienced an allergic reaction to your cancer treatment.
- Avoid drinking or eating if you are having diarrhea. Discuss an appropriate diet with a nutritionist or dietitian.
- Wait to inform your doctor of side effects; most can be treated, so intervening promptly is critical to continue your anti-cancer treatment.

in the mouth. In other cases, people with the so-called paraneoplastic syndromes with stomach or lung cancer may have darkened, thick skin in the armpits or groin. Some colorectal and urinary cancers may cause excess growth of fine hair all over the body. It's important to be aware of these changes and discuss them with your doctor to find their cause and begin effective treatments as soon as possible.

Skin problems may result from anti-cancer medications and radiation. For people living with cancer, skin problems that result from treatment are among the most important side effects. Chemotherapy and ra-

DID YOU KNOW?

Anti-cancer treatments that affect the skin are not only a common but an expected consequence of the way treatments work—that is, by blocking the growth of cells.

diation will attack and destroy fast-growing cancer cells. But these treatments can't tell the difference between fast-growing cancer cells and fast-growing healthy cells in the skin, mouth, hair roots, or nails. The severity of effects in the skin depends on several factors: the type and dose of chemotherapy or radiation used; how often it is received; the way in which treatment is given (orally or through a vein); other diseases (heart conditions and diabetes are especially important) or medications (such as those that suppress the immune system); body weight, age, and gender; the severity and type of cancer; and a person's activity level. Although these side effects may be mildly annoying when they occur for a short time, many of them can last for weeks or months, affecting a person's quality of life and in some cases even health. Radiation treatment, for example, can irritate the skin and may lead to both short-term and long-lasting skin effects, even many years later.

Over the past decades, scientists have developed effective anti-cancer medications known as targeted therapies. These treatments differ from chemotherapy in that they are designed to block specific molecules that direct cancer cells to grow and spread. As a result, targeted therapies tend to spare healthy cells in the body and cause fewer side effects than conventional chemotherapy (such as nausea and vomiting, weakness, hair loss, and serious infections). Despite these advantages, targeted therapies have unexpectedly resulted in many side effects affecting the skin—most of which are treatable.

Targeted therapies are given orally or intravenously (IV—through a vein) and are used to treat many cancers including those of the colon, lungs, breasts, head and neck, kidneys, thyroid, skin, stomach, pancreas, and brain. Because targeted therapies affect molecules essential to the growth of skin, hair, and nails, they lead to inflammation of the skin, rash, tenderness, itching, dryness, as well as nail and hair changes.

It's important to note that targeted therapies are usually given for many months or even indefinitely, so side effects that may seem unimportant at first can become bothersome after a while. That is why it is so important to treat any skin problem early on—even when it is mild—and prevent it when possible. When you are examined for a rash during cancer treatment, be sure that your health care team is aware of all the medicines you are taking. That includes any drugs used for other reasons or those given to prevent and treat other side effects of chemotherapy.

Although rashes that occur during cancer treatment are seldom life-threatening, diagnosing and treating a rash yourself, with over-the-counter medicines you may already have, is usually not a good idea. In some cases, the rash may get worse or result in a skin infection, leading to changes or interruptions in your cancer treatment. Proper evaluation of a rash requires a visit to an oncologist or dermatologist familiar with cancer treatments and their effect on skin. If treated early and appropriately, most rashes improve and are short-lived (see Chapter 2).

Cancer surgery can scar the skin. Once the integrity of the skin is altered, as with surgery, a scar will form. Scarring from surgery for breast, thyroid, sarcomas, or head and neck cancer, for instance, may affect patients psychologically or alter their ability to function physically. Ideally, the scars should be as small as possible and oriented in a specific way, so they are difficult to see and feel.

Stem cell transplants for blood cancers such as leukemias, lymphomas, and myelomas can lead to many skin changes, especially a rash. This type of rash often starts on the head and trunk and may gradually spread to the entire body. People living with transplants may also experience slower hair and nail growth.

Because some of the newer cancer treatments are so effective and cause fewer problems with infections, nausea, or vomiting, side effects of the skin, hair, and nails are receiving more attention. Effects of cancer treatments on the skin are either acute (within hours or days) or late (months to years after the end of treatment). Late effects are important to monitor because

DID YOU KNOW?

Most of the side effects of anti-cancer treatments are known by the time medications are approved for use. Severe skin side effects to chemotherapies are extremely rare.

they can affect a person's quality of life for a long time if they are not addressed. Be sure to talk with your doctor or nurse about any symptoms you experience. The good news is that most dermatologic side effects during treatment are mild or moderate in severity, and they can be treated effectively.

THINGS TO REMEMBER

- The skin is the largest organ in the body with many functions, including protection, temperature regulation, and the formation of hair and nails.

- The skin, hair and nails are constantly renewing and changing, making them susceptible to chemotherapy and radiation, which attack fast-growing cells.

- Skin changes can sometimes be the first sign of an underlying cancer. This can occur in people with inherited family cancer syndromes or with paraneoplastic syndromes.

- Cancer itself can affect the skin in different ways: by occurring directly in the skin; by spreading from other organs to the skin; or by releasing chemicals that result in rashes or growths on the skin.

- Dermatologic side effects are amongst the most frequent and unexpected side effects. There are more than 52 different skin, hair, and nail side effects that may develop from cancer treatments (surgery, radiation, anti-cancer drugs).

- Cancers of the skin are more common and more serious in people living with leukemias, lymphomas, or stem cell transplants. Skin cancers may also result from certain anti-cancer treatments.

- Dermatologic side effects to chemotherapies are usually not allergies, which allows for treatments to continue.

- Type and dose of medications, severity of cancer, and overall health are some of the many factors that may predispose some people to dermatologic side effects.

- Most dermatologic side effects are manageable, so that people can maintain their quality of life and continue their cancer treatments.

- Life-threatening skin side effects to chemotherapy are extremely rare.

CHAPTER 2

All Rashes Are Not Created Equal

You have probably heard from your oncologist or nurse that the medicine you are about to receive may cause a rash. Although rashes to chemotherapy or targeted therapies are usually not severe, they can be uncomfortable and in some cases may lead to your doctor decreasing or changing your treatment. So it's important to tell your health care team as soon as you notice a rash or other types of skin changes. Your health care team can then take the right steps to treat the rash and ensure that treatment continues uninterrupted.

In this chapter, you'll learn about:

- Medications that cause rash
- What different types of rash look like
- Ways to prevent and treat rash
- How to tell the difference between inconsequential and life-threatening rashes

Aside from the side effects most often associated with chemotherapy—tiredness, nausea and vomiting, diarrhea, infections, and so on—people receiving any anti-cancer treatment can develop a rash. Most symptoms associated with a rash caused by chemotherapy or targeted therapies (discussed in more detail in the following pages) gradually go away after treatment ends. In time, healthy skin cells grow normally again. How long this process takes depends on factors such as age, gender, overall health, type and severity of the cancer, type of cancer medications, and whether the

DID YOU KNOW?

Rash is a name given to many different conditions that affect the skin. It usually presents with red or purple spots or bumps and may be itchy or painful.

rash is treated appropriately. Although some medications can cause long-lasting changes to certain organs in the body (such as the heart), most people have no long-term skin problems from these treatments (as opposed to rashes related to radiation or to stem cell transplants, which may be long-lasting).

Medicines That May Cause a Rash

Aside from chemotherapy, a number of other medications given during the course of cancer treatments can also cause rashes. The table below lists the most common examples of medications that are used by people undergoing treatment.

Timing (of Rash Onset) Is Everything

Knowing when a rash appears can give your doctor many clues as to what is causing it, what needs to be done to treat it, and the implications for continued cancer treatment. With most anti-cancer medications, a rash appears within the first two months after beginning treatment. Rashes that begin during this time are usually treatable, and anti-cancer treatments can

Medicines That Can Cause Rash
Antibiotics (penicillin, sulfa-based antibiotics)
Anti-seizure medications (phenytoin, valproic acid)
Anti-pain medications (codeine, hydromorphone, oxycodone)
Anti-inflammatories (ibuprofen, naproxen)
Blood pressure and heart medicines (captopril, hydrochlorothiazide)
Anti-uric acid (or gout) medicines (allopurinol)
Medicines used to treat side effects to chemotherapy such as nausea and vomiting (ondansetron, aprepitant) or diarrhea (loperamide, octreotide)
Corticosteroids (such as dexamethasone, prednisone)
Medicines for low levels of blood cells (such as filgrastim or pegfilgrastim)
Blood thinners (enoxaparin, warfarin)

be continued. It's important to keep in mind that most rashes are a direct effect of the medicine on your skin, which means that it is not an allergic reaction. Rashes that appear more than three months after starting an anti-cancer treatment are probably not related to it, and so the current medications may continue. In these cases, it may be a skin condition unrelated to cancer or its treatment. Nonetheless, it should be treated so that it doesn't affect your overall health and well-being.

On the other hand, when a rash starts appearing within minutes or hours of starting chemotherapy or a targeted therapy, or even within the first day the drug is received, it could be an allergic reaction, which can be a serious threat to a person's health. In such cases, the drug must be stopped. If you are diagnosed as being allergic to a medication, it is important to inform all of your doctors, so your medical records can be updated. Information about allergies should be included in a medication list or displayed on a necklace or bracelet.

Whether a rash appears immediately or after a few days, it is important to keep track of when the skin changes or other symptoms were noticed so you can inform your doctor. With so many things going on, it's easy to forget. Many people say that keeping a diary is extremely helpful to accurately document when symptoms develop or change. Also, taking photos of the rash may be helpful, as it tends to change. Ask a friend or family member to take a photo of the rash with a camera or cell phone. Make sure you have good lighting and focus. I always recommend taking photos from different angles: one photo from far away (that shows the upper, mid, or lower body), another directly showing the specific body area (such as the face, chest, or arm), and one close up (about 6 inches away). These views will help your doctor determine what kind of rash it is.

When It Comes to Rash, Appearance Matters

What a rash looks like is very important, as it will help your doctor diagnose whether it is caused by your

> **DID YOU KNOW?**
> A rash can be caused by medications (chemotherapies or others), can be part of a skin condition related or unrelated to cancer, or can occur as a result of an infection.

Q My doctor said that a rash from targeted therapy means the medicine is working. She prescribed a corticosteroid cream and an antibiotic, which have made it better. I'm happy that the rash has improved, but does this mean my targeted therapy is not working anymore?

A With some of the so-called targeted therapies (bortezomib, cetuximab, erlotinib, gefitinib, and panitumumab), development of a rash means the medication is having a greater anti-cancer effect. However, people who don't develop a rash can still benefit from these medicines. And for those who do develop a rash, treating it will not reduce the beneficial effect of the targeted treatment. In fact, managing the rash prevents discomfort and reduces the chance of having to change or stop your targeted therapy.

anti-cancer medicine and in some cases which medicine (if several are being taken at the same time) is the culprit. How do doctors distinguish between different types of rashes? It's like completing a puzzle in which many different features come together to reach a diagnosis. First, the basic component of a rash must be determined, and this is what doctors call a *lesion*. A lesion is a change in the skin, and a group of lesions forms a rash.

When doctors examine a rash, they evaluate its appearance (whether it is raised [bumpy] or flat); its color (red, purple, yellow, or white); its shape (round, oval, or appearing as lines); whether it is dry, flaky, or moist; how much of the body's skin is affected; the location (face, trunk, or legs); and whether the rash is associated with itching, pain, or nothing at all. These characteristics help determine the cause of the rash—a drug, an infection, or a specific skin condition—so that the best treatment can be chosen.

Managing Rashes: An Overview

Before beginning chemotherapy or a targeted therapy, it is important to become familiar with each medication you are taking and its possible side effects. Ask

The "Good News" About Rash From Targeted Therapies

A few years ago, doctors initially noticed that people with colon cancer who received the targeted therapy cetuximab and had a rash did better than those who did not develop the rash. The more severe the rash, the better their cancer responded to the medicine. This unusual benefit from a rash has only been seen in those cancers treated with some of the targeted treatments, such as bortezomib, cetuximab, erlotinib gefitinib, and panitumumab.

This link between rash and effectiveness of treatment has not been seen with conventional chemotherapy.

Although the rash may be a good sign, it is important to treat it, so it doesn't get to a point where it will affect well-being or result in a change in the dose of the medication. Studies have also shown that treating or even preventing the rash will not decrease the effectiveness of these medicines.

your oncologist whether you are likely to experience a rash with your particular medication and what you should do if one appears. It's a good idea to keep your health care team's contact information handy. As soon as you begin to notice any skin side effects, contact your doctor or nurse so you can get treatment and avoid more serious symptoms. Here are some other things to remember:

While you are receiving cancer treatments, it's important to protect yourself against the sun, since many medications (chemotherapies, targeted therapies, antibiotics, and antifungals) increase your sensitivity to sunlight. Use a sunscreen with a high sun protection factor (SPF). Ideally, the SPF should be at least 15, and the sunscreen should contain zinc oxide. It should be applied every two hours or more frequently if you are sweating or swimming. Make sure you use more than half a teaspoon each on the head and neck area, half a teaspoon for the right and the left arm, and more than one teaspoon each for your front, back, and each leg. See Chapter 10, "Sun Safety," for more details.

Q Are there any foods that can affect a rash caused by anti-cancer medicines?

A No foods consistently cause a rash to get better or worse during treatment. However, if your medication is to be taken orally, make sure that you follow directions. Some need to be taken with food, such as capecitabine. Others, such as abiraterone, deferasirox, eltrombopag, erlotinib, lapatinib, nilotinib, sorafenib, and voriconazole, need to be taken on an empty stomach. With other medications, such as sunitinib and everolimus, it doesn't matter whether they are taken with or without food.

Q Are there any vitamin or herbal supplements I can take to prevent or treat a rash during treatment?

A No vitamin or herbal supplements have been shown to prevent or treat a rash from any type of anti-cancer treatment. Usually, only calcium and vitamin D supplements are allowed during treatment. Consult with your oncologist, since some supplements may affect the effectiveness of treatments and even liver function. Information on vitamins can be found at the Office of Dietary Supplements at the National Institutes of Health (www.ods.od.nih.gov). For more information on herbal supplements, visit Memorial Sloan-Kettering Cancer Center's website (www.mskcc.org/aboutherbs).

Before using any over-the-counter medications, talk with your doctor or nurse. It's important to note that rashes associated with anti-cancer medicines will usually not respond to over-the-counter medications. Treating the rash with prescription-strength medications will be more effective and will allow the anti-cancer therapy to continue. When washing the skin, avoid using anti-acne skin products, such as those containing alcohol, benzoyl peroxide, salicylic acid, or vitamin A-type creams (retinoids), unless prescribed by your doctor. These products can dry your skin.

Be gentle with your skin. As soon as you begin receiving chemotherapy, targeted therapies, or radiation therapy, use a mild, fragrance-free soap when bathing or showering; avoid soaps with strong scents.

Important Information About Rashes to Share With Your Doctor or Nurse

- When did it start, and how fast is it spreading?
- What is the shape of the lesions?
- Which parts of the body are affected?
- Is it flat or raised?
- What color is it?
- Is it scaly or smooth?
- Is it dry or moist?
- Is it itchy or painful?
- Are there blisters or pus bumps?
- Is there anything that makes it better or worse?
- Have you used anything to treat it (including over-the-counter products)?

Questions to Ask Your Doctor About Rash

- Is the rash related to my anti-cancer treatment?
- Is it an allergy that will prevent me from getting more treatment?
- Is a skin sample (biopsy) or culture needed? If so, will it help determine what to do next?
- May I continue my cancer treatment with this rash?
- What topical or oral medicines should I use?
- Is it likely to reappear? If so, is there anything that can be done to prevent that from happening?

It's best to avoid long, hot showers or baths, which make rashes worse; use lukewarm water instead. Do not use loofahs or sponges to clean or scrub, as they are loaded with infection-causing germs. Apply a moisturizer to the skin within 15 minutes of showering or bathing. Hypoallergenic moisturizers that do not have perfumes or preservatives are best, but remember that hypoallergenic products still have some chemicals in them that you may be allergic to. One brand considered to be truly free of chemicals and substances known to cause allergies or irritate skin is Vanicream.

Q I'm getting a rash, and I would like to be seen by a dermatologist. How do I find this type of specialist close to where I live?

A There are more than 80,000 dermatology practices in the United States. You can ask your oncologist for a referral or search in the American Academy of Dermatology website (www.aad.org). Make sure you bring a list of all the medicines you are receiving from your oncologist or any other doctor. If possible, bring a copy of your records and your oncologist's name and phone number. Before your dermatology appointment, prepare a list of questions and bring a piece of paper or notebook to write down the answers. It's always a good idea to bring along a friend or relative for support and to help keep track of the information.

How Rash Is Treated: The Three I's

For most medication-induced rashes, choosing a treatment is based on stopping the three I's:

- Inflammation
- Itching
- Infections

Soothing Skin Inflammation in Rashes

Skin inflammation is visible as redness, bumps, or swelling and can be controlled with the use of oral or topical corticosteroids or antibiotics. Most rashes to anti-cancer medicines have inflammation as the main feature, which is associated with skin pain or itching. Corticosteroids are a type of hormone normally produced by the body that suppresses inflammation and the symptoms associated with it (pain or itching). Corticosteroids are also produced in a laboratory for use as a medication in creams, ointments, pills, or injections.

For several reasons, corticosteroids have a bad reputation: athletes use anabolic steroids to illegally enhance performance (a different type of steroid than the one used for medical purposes), and corticosteroids tend to weaken the immune system and bones. They also alter mood and make people lose sleep and gain weight. These side effects occur at very high doses or when corticosteroids are taken for a long time. When used correctly, they are extremely effective. It's worth noting that corticosteroids have been used for medical purposes for more than 40 years, so their side effects are well understood and mostly reversible once they have been stopped. There are many different types of medicated corticosteroids, with varying strengths and duration of action, both of which will determine when and where in the body they are used, as well as how frequently they need to be used and for how long.

Topical Corticosteroids

Hydrocortisone A number of over-the-counter brands (Cortizone-10, Hytone) are available. Considered to be low strength, hydrocortisone has few side effects and can be used safely on the face, groin, or under the arms for weeks to months at a time.

Triamcinolone A medium-strength corticosteroid, triamcinolone is good for rashes on the trunk or limbs. It can also be used safely for weeks to months at a time. For short periods (a few days or up to a couple of weeks), it can be used on the face, groin, or under the arms.

Fluocinonide One of the strongest and most effective corticosteroids is fluocinonide. Sometimes it is needed for a severe rash but should not be used for more than one week at a time. It also available as a solution or a foam, which is easy to apply to rashes on the scalp or other hairy areas.

Clobetasol The strongest of all corticosteroids is clobetasol. No more than 50 grams (about two ounces) of clobetasol can be used in one week, and it can be used for mouth sores from everolimus and temsirolimus.

Oral or Intravenous Corticosteroids

Oral corticosteroids need to be prescribed by your doctor; they are even more effective than topical steroids. The most commonly prescribed include dexamethasone, methylprednisolone, and prednisone. Dexamethasone is frequently given before certain chemotherapies (cisplatin, docetaxel, paclitaxel) to prevent allergic reactions, nausea, and vomiting. When used for a rash, oral corticosteroids are usually given as pills or tablets for one to two weeks. If you need to use these drugs for a longer time, your doctor will likely reduce the dose gradually over a few days or weeks, so that the rash does not rebound and your body's naturally produced corticosteroids have time to adjust.

Improving Itch

One of the most common (and most bothersome) symptoms associated with rashes to chemotherapy or targeted therapies is itching. Itching can be treated with topical medicines when it's not severe or when it's localized to one part of the body. Oral medicines are used when the itching is so severe that it affects sleep or the ability to go about daily activities, or when it is so widespread that it's not practical to apply a topical medicine. In some cases, even if there is no visible rash, your doctor will prescribe oral or topical corticosteroids to control itch. For more detailed information on itch and treatment options, see Chapter 4, "How to Stop the Itching."

Topical Anti-Itch Medications

Menthol Included in many anti-itch and anti-pain products (Gold Bond Anti-Itch Lotion or Cream, Sarna Original Anti-Itch Lotion, Eucerin Calming Itch-Relief Treatment), menthol provides a cooling sensation. However, people living with cancer who have a heightened sense of smell may find it unpleasant.

Pramoxine An anesthetic that "numbs" the skin to any sensation (Prax, Sarna Sensitive Lotion, Aveeno Anti-Itch Cream or Concentrated Lotion, Gold Bond Anti-Itch Lotion or Cream, Caladryl Anti-Itch Lotion). Although pramoxine is safe and effective, the benefit is often short-lived, requiring frequent applications.

Use Topical Corticosteroids With Caution

Topical corticosteroids are very effective at improving rashes, skin itch, and inflammation. However, when strong corticosteroids such as clobetasol or fluocinonide are used continuously for several months or more in the same area, they can cause irreversible side effects— skin thinning, stretch marks, dilated blood vessels, discoloration, and infections. Even less strong corticosteroids such as triamcinolone can cause these side effects when used on the face, groin, or armpits for a long time. So always look at your skin for signs of side effects, and ask your doctor for specific instructions.

Lidocaine A stronger numbing medicine than pramoxine is lidocaine, or the combination of lidocaine and prilocaine (EMLA), obtained with a doctor's prescription. Lidocaine must be used carefully, because it can be absorbed in the body. A numbing patch is available for people with itch or pain from shingles or other intense, localized forms of pain or itch.

Doxepin An antihistamine cream applied four times a day for several weeks, doxepin can also be taken as a pill. A prescription is needed for doxepin, since its application over large body areas results in drowsiness in about 25 percent of people.

Oral Anti-Itch Medications

Cetirizine, fexofenadine, and loratadine These over-the-counter antihistamines help with itch for up to 24 hours. They do not cause significant drowsiness in most people.

Diphenhydramine and hydroxyzine These antihistamines are more effective at controlling itch but also cause more drowsiness. If drowsiness becomes a problem, take cetirizine, fexofenadine, or loratadine during the day and one of these stronger antihistamines at night (which will also help you sleep better). Topical diphenhydramine is not recommended by dermatologists. It's not very effective, and people can become allergic to it.

DID YOU KNOW?

The ingredient camphor is sometimes added to anti-itch products to produce a cooling sensation. Another way of achieving this effect is by keeping your anti-itch products in the refrigerator.

Doxepin This antihistamine also has antidepressant properties and is very effective against itch. It is usually used after other antihistamines have been tried. Doxepin also causes significant drowsiness, so it would be a good option for people who are having trouble sleeping, though it must be used with caution in those taking antidepressant medications.

Gabapentin and pregabalin These medications are used to relieve pain. They work by modulating, or changing, the sensitivity of nerve endings. These medications must be adjusted if the kidneys are not working properly and can also cause some drowsiness and swelling of the legs.

Specific causes of itch require unique treatments. For example, in people living with the bone marrow disease polycythemia vera, taking 300 mg a day of aspirin can improve itching. Also, the anti-nausea medicine **aprepitant** has been shown to help ease the itch associated with targeted therapies, skin lymphomas, and other types of cancer. In cases where itch is severe and not improved with medicines, doctors may recommend **phototherapy**, also known as UV light therapy. This type of treatment is often used for skin conditions such as psoriasis and eczema. It requires a special type of artificial UV light at a dermatologist's office. The light blunts the skin's immune system, reducing the number of cells that promote itch.

Infections: Fighting Germs as a Way of Treating Rashes

In up to one third of people treated with anti-cancer medications and developing a rash, skin infections can occur as a result of the skin being damaged from the rash. Antibiotics are often used to manage skin infections, but sometimes they are used even when there is no apparent skin infection. There are two reasons for this: First, once your skin has a rash, bacteria that normally live on the surface of your skin can grow quickly and cause disease. Second, some antibiotics are thought to have an anti-inflammatory effect on the skin, thus helping relieve rashes. Your doctor will decide which antibiotic needs to be used, based on several factors such as the location of the rash on the body, potential side effects, and whether it will interact with chemotherapy. Most likely, your doctor will also obtain a culture to identify the germ causing the infection and which antibiotic would be most effective. It usually takes three to five days for the results of a culture to come back, but before that, your doctor will probably prescribe an antibiotic that is likely to be effective.

Topical Antibiotics

Clindamycin One of the most commonly used topical antibiotics, clindamycin is effective against most bacteria known to cause skin infections. It is available as a gel, lotion, or foam; the foam is good for hairy areas, such as the scalp.

Mupirocin A good antibiotic for a common skin germ, *Staphylococcus aureus,* and even the much talked about MRSA, a type of staphylococcus that resists common antibiotics. Available as a cream or an ointment, mupirocin is also effective when crusting (sometimes with bleeding) appears inside the nose, which is usually a sign of bacterial overgrowth resulting in a condition called nasal vestibulitis. When skin infections occur frequently, doctors try to get rid of as much skin bacteria as possible in a process called decolonization. In such cases, mupirocin is applied twice daily on the armpits, groin, and inside the nose, and bleach baths (one cup of bleach in a bathtub full of water) or the use of a chlorhexidine wash in the shower is recommended to reduce skin infections and the amount of bacteria in body areas harboring high concentrations of disease-causing germs.

Silver sulfadiazine Effective against many different bacteria and yeast (has what doctors call a "broad spectrum" of action), silver sulfadiazine normally is used for burn victims. People with an allergy to sulfa-type antibiotics should avoid it. It is commonly used for skin that is very painful or sensitive, such as radiation-induced rash and skin infections, as it doesn't sting or burn when applied. Also, silver sulfadiazine is a good antibiotic to use in the groin, since that area harbors many different types of bacteria.

Oral or Intravenous Antibiotics

There are dozens of antibiotics that can be used to fight infection, but here are some of the most commonly used by dermatologists.

Doxycycline and minocycline These medications are dermatologists' favorite antibiotics, as they have been tried and true for many skin infections and are proven to be effective for many skin conditions including acne and rosacea due to their potential anti-inflammatory properties. Major side effects are sensitivity to the sun (doxycycline), vertigo (minocycline), nausea, and diarrhea, so they are better tolerated if taken with food. These antibiotics are also effective at preventing the acne-like rash from the targeted therapies cetuximab, erlotinib, gefitinib, panitumumab, and vandetanib.

Trimethoprim-sulfamethoxazole This commonly used antibiotic destroys many different types of bacteria. About three percent of people are allergic to its sulfa component. It also causes sensitivity to the sun and, rarely, can affect the blood. This antibiotic must be taken with caution by people receiving chemotherapy, as sometimes it can affect cells in the blood.

Ciprofloxacin and levofloxacin These antibiotics also widely used because they are effective against many different types of bacteria. They must be used carefully by people with a history of heart or tendon/joint problems (especially if receiving oral corticosteroids at the same time).

A Rash By Any Other Name

Most rashes are not serious and will not affect your course of treatment, so it is important to understand the different types of rash. In most people receiving chemotherapy or targeted therapy, rashes result from a direct effect of the medication in the skin. Along with the destruction of cancer cells, these medicines also damage skin cells. Most types of rashes from cancer medications are not associated with signs of an allergy (shortness of breath; fainting; throat tightness; swelling of the eyelids

Grading the Severity of a Rash

Determining how severe a rash is will depend on several factors, including how much of the skin is affected (the skin on the palm of the hand represents about one percent of the entire area of the body's skin surface) and whether the rash affects emotional or physical well-being.

Grade 1 (Mild) A mild rash that is usually not associated with pain, itching, or burning and does not always require treatment. Grade 1 rashes usually cover less than 10 percent of the skin (the face, scalp, and neck are about 10 percent of the skin).

Grade 2 (Moderate) This severity of rash is probably the most common and is usually associated with pain, itching, burning, or some other discomfort. Treatments include creams, ointments, or pills, and the anti-cancer medication causing it can usually be continued. By the time a rash is grade 2 or worse, it can affect a person's self-esteem. The rash may also affect a person's ability to prepare meals, shop, use the telephone, or handle money. Grade 2 rashes usually cover 10 to 30 percent of the skin on the body (the entire face, chest, and upper back are approximately 20 percent of the skin).

Grade 3 (Severe) Rashes this severe are not that common. Grade 3 rashes are usually itchy or painful and may result in skin infections that require oral antibiotics or admission to the hospital. A grade 3 rash may affect a person's ability to bathe, get dressed, eat, use the toilet, or take medications. Grade 3 rashes usually cover more than 30 percent of the skin (the face, entire back and chest, and stomach are more than 30 percent) and will often require an interruption or reduction of the anti-cancer treatment.

Grade 4 (Very Severe) Rashes this severe are extremely rare. They are life-threatening and require urgent treatments (intravenous medicines or surgical procedures). At this grade, anti-cancer medications need to be stopped, sometimes indefinitely, and another medication is then used.

Q I had itching that was probably related to chemotherapy, but it's gone now, thanks to the antihistamine my doctor prescribed. I don't want to take medicines if I don't have to, so do I still need to take this pill?

A Since itch is a symptom, rather than a disease, it does not require continued treatment if it is no longer present. Once the itch goes away, you can stop taking or applying anti-itch medicines. Just use them as needed. However, if there is a rash associated with the itch, it's important to treat the rash also. If your doctor is recommending antihistamines to prevent allergies to a chemotherapy, you should continue to use them as indicated.

Q My doctor recommended that I apply an anti-itch cream to my back, but I can't reach that area. Are there any tips on how to apply creams on the back?

A If no one is available to help, you can use a special applicator such as the Lotion Applicator Back Brush from Bed Bath and Beyond, Roll Easy Lotion Applicator (made by The Wright Stuff, Inc.), Roll-a-Lotion Applicator, Kingsley Lotion Applicator, or Earth Therapeutics Lotion Applicator. They are available at pharmacies, retail or surgical supply stores, or online at Amazon.com (www.amazon.com).

DID YOU KNOW?
For people who have difficulty swallowing pills, many antibiotics are also available as a liquid that can be either swallowed or administered through a stomach tube.

or lips; welts; or sores in the mouth, eyes, or genitals). Armed with this knowledge, doctors can act to improve a rash and avoid the need to stop or change the anti-cancer treatment. Overall, how severe a rash is will help your oncologist determine how to treat it and whether to change the dose, frequency, or type of medication. (See the box on page 25 on grading the severity of a rash.)

Non-allergic Rash This is the most common type of rash and is caused by many anti-cancer medications that have a direct effect on the skin (as opposed to triggering an allergy). It is not life-threatening and is usually expected in up to two thirds of people after they have begun receiving a targeted therapy, appearing after several weeks of beginning treatment in most individuals. The important thing is that anti-cancer treatments can usually be continued if this type of rash is treated or is not severe. Unlike allergic rashes, this type of rash improves with prescription-strength creams or pills, even when the anti-cancer treatment continues.

Allergic and/or Serious Rash Most cancer treatments will not cause allergic or serious rashes. Although very rare, an allergic or serious rash is unpredictable and can be life-threatening. Allergic rashes usually appear within minutes to hours of starting treatment or within the first few cycles. Culprit medications usually need to be stopped. Fortunately, in most cases, oncologists have other medications they can use. A consultation with an allergist is a good idea, since there are skin tests that may help confirm the problem drug, especially if it is one of the platinum drugs (carboplatin, cisplatin, or oxaliplatin). In some cases, if the oncologist decides that chemotherapy must continue despite an allergic rash, they can be given in the hospital under the careful supervision of nurses, doctors, and allergy specialists.

Anti-cancer Medications That May Cause Allergic Rashes

Asparaginase	Estramustine	Oprelvekin
Alemtuzumab	Etoposide	Paclitaxel
Bexarotene	Filgrastim	Pemetrexed
Bicalutamide	Gemcitabine	Procarbazine
Bleomycin	Goserelin	Rituximab
Carboplatin	Ibritumomab	Temozolomide
Cetuximab	Ifosfamide	Teniposide
Cisplatin	Interferon	Temsirolimus
Cladribine	Interleukin-2	Thiotepa
Cyclophosphamide	Irinotecan	Tositumomab
Cytarabine	Medroxyprogesterone	Trastuzumab
Docetaxel	Mitoxantrone	Vincristine
Epoetin alfa	Octreotide	Vinorelbine

Q If I develop a rash during treatment, how do I know if it is an allergic or serious rash?

A Although a serious allergic rash is rare, warning signs include:

- Difficulty breathing or throat tightness
- Passing out or fainting
- Uncontrollable diarrhea or sneezing
- Swelling of the lips or eyelids
- Painful blisters in the mouth and genitals
- Severe abdominal or back pain
- Hives or itching all over the body

When these signs are present, doctors may decide to stop the anti-cancer treatment and give anti-allergy medications through a vein. In special cases where it is necessary to continue the same anti-cancer treatment despite the allergy, doctors may give it in smaller doses under supervision in the hospital, along with anti-allergy medications, in a process known as desensitization.

DID YOU KNOW?

With targeted therapies, a rash may be an indicator that the medication is working.

Location and Look of a Rash

Both the location of the rash on your body and what it looks like are key to successful diagnosis and treatment. Be sure to tell your health care team these details about your rash.

Red Bumps and Flaking on the Scalp

The scalp is an area of skin that has one of the highest concentrations of hair and blood vessels, so medications that affect hair follicles or blood vessels can lead to a scalp rash. In particular, cyclophosphamide, docetaxel, paclitaxel, and sorafenib may cause itching and sometimes a painful, bumpy rash. This rash is treated with topical or oral antibiotics or corticosteroid foams, lotions, or shampoos. With sorafenib, the scalp may become very sensitive, making it difficult to comb or wash the hair or even rest the head on a pillow. Corticosteroids are beneficial, either topically or orally.

When caused by an anti-cancer medication, scalp flaking is usually not caused by dryness but rather in-

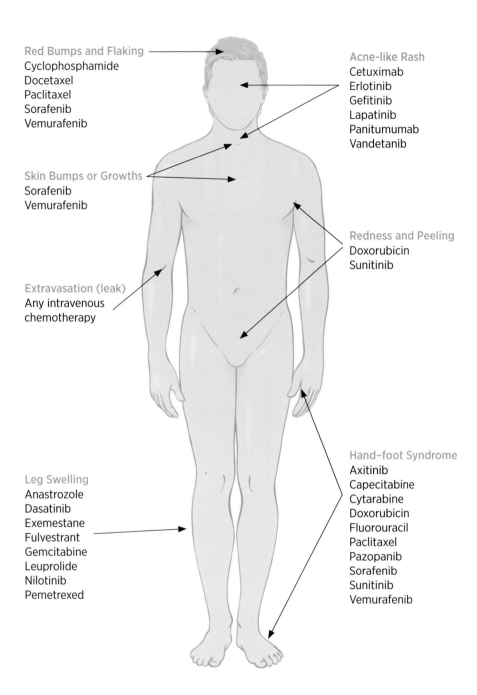

Red Bumps and Flaking
Cyclophosphamide
Docetaxel
Paclitaxel
Sorafenib
Vemurafenib

Skin Bumps or Growths
Sorafenib
Vemurafenib

Extravasation (leak)
Any intravenous
chemotherapy

Leg Swelling
Anastrozole
Dasatinib
Exemestane
Fulvestrant
Gemcitabine
Leuprolide
Nilotinib
Pemetrexed

Acne-like Rash
Cetuximab
Erlotinib
Gefitinib
Lapatinib
Panitumumab
Vandetanib

Redness and Peeling
Doxorubicin
Sunitinib

Hand–foot Syndrome
Axitinib
Capecitabine
Cytarabine
Doxorubicin
Fluorouracil
Paclitaxel
Pazopanib
Sorafenib
Sunitinib
Vemurafenib

LOCATIONS AND MEDICATIONS
The location and appearance of rash on the body will give clues as to which medication is the cause. Here are some of the most common locations and presentations of anti-cancer therapy-induced rashes and the medications that cause them. Most other rashes (red bumps on the body, blisters, and hives or welts) could be caused by almost any medication, including those not specifically used against cancer.

Medications That May Lead to Scalp or Face Rash

Affecting mostly the scalp:

Cyclophosphamide	Sorafenib
Docetaxel	Paclitaxel

Affecting the scalp and face:

Cetuximab	Panitumumab
Erlotinib	Sorafenib
Gefitinib	Vandetanib

flammation and shedding of dead skin cells. There is no need to avoid washing your scalp or hair if this occurs, since shampooing will not make it worse. In cases unrelated to medications, this flaking can result from an increased growth of a yeast, which causes dandruff. In some situations, such as with brain or neurologic cancers, dandruff may become severe, resulting in a very flaky scalp. For this severe dandruff, shampoos containing zinc pyrithione (DHS Shampoo and Conditioners), ketoconazole, or ciclopirox will reduce the scaling and inflammation. If there is itching, topical corticosteroids are helpful.

Red, Bumpy Rash on the Trunk and Extremities

Resembling the measles, this is probably one of the most common types of rash. It may be caused by any type of chemotherapy or targeted therapy, most commonly docetaxel, ipilimumab, paclitaxel, sorafenib, trastuzumab, and vemurafenib. Known as morbilliform by doctors, it contains both red spots (macules) and bumps (papules). The spots are usually bright red, pink, or salmon-colored, and the skin may feel hot, burning, or itchy. The rash appears to begin near the center of the body (the chest, back, and stomach) and then travels to the arms and legs; the face may be spared. This rash usually occurs up to one month after

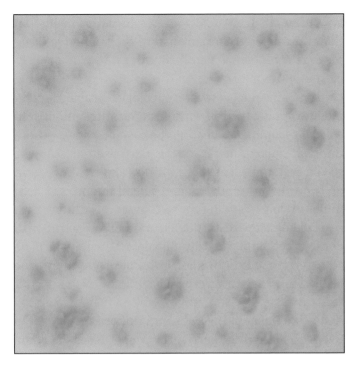

RED, BUMPY RASH
Resembling the measles, this common rash begins near the center of the body and then travels to the arms and legs.

treatment has been initiated, but it is most likely to appear within the first ten days of treatment.

Most of the time, this type of rash is not a problem if treated effectively, so the anti-cancer therapy can continue. But if any of the symptoms listed in the box below appear, see your doctor right away. They

Signs That a Rash May Be Serious

- Swelling of the lips or eyelids
- Sneezing, welts, and intense itching all over the body
- Fever, uncontrollable diarrhea or sneezing, and abdominal or back pain
- Difficulty breathing, tightness in the throat, or fainting

are potential signs of an allergy, which may mean that the anti-cancer treatment has to be stopped, so that anti-rash medicines (antihistamines and/or cortico-steroids) can take effect.

When the rash is severe, oncologists usually recommend stopping the responsible medication until it subsides. I recommend treating the rash promptly, even if the rash-causing medication is decreased or stopped, so the rash improves more quickly and treatment can be restarted promptly. A good rule of thumb is to continue treating the rash for one to two weeks after it has resolved or after restarting chemotherapy, so the rash doesn't "rebound." Usually, oncologists will restart the anti-cancer medications at a lower dose after they have been withheld for a severe rash.

Acne-like Rash on the Face and Upper Body

Between 50 and 90 percent of people receiving some targeted therapies experience a rash that looks like acne, affecting the face, scalp, neck, chest, and upper body. The rash usually occurs within two weeks after the start of treatment and may improve over the next few months, making the first two months the most difficult in terms of dealing with this rash.

This rash may look like acne, but it is not acne, as it also affects the scalp, and it itches and hurts in most

Anti-cancer Medications That May Cause Acne-like Rash

Cetuximab	Lapatinib
Corticosteroids	Paclitaxel
Cyclophosphamide	Panitumumab
Docetaxel	Sorafenib
Erlotinib	Sunitinib
Everolimus	Temsirolimus
Gefitinib	Vandetanib

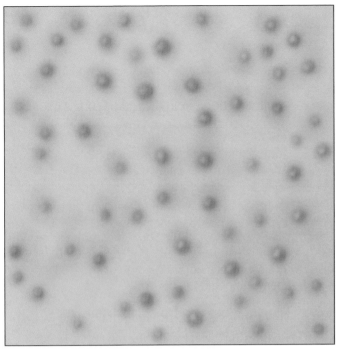

ACNE-LIKE RASH
Often associated with the use of targeted therapies, this rash looks like acne and affects the face, scalp, neck, chest, and upper body. However, it is not acne, since it hurts, itches, and spreads beyond the face.

DID YOU KNOW?

Scars from acne, or acne-like rash are not caused by "picking", but rather by the inflammation in the skin causing permanent damage. Hence the reason for preventing or treating acne or acne-like rash when possible.

people. The box on the opposite page lists anti-cancer medications that may cause this acne-like rash.

Acne-like rashes tend to be mild to moderate in most people, but, in some cases, they can be severe and uncomfortable. Because targeted therapies usually need to be taken for many months or indefinitely, it's more difficult to tolerate a "mild" to "moderate" rash when it lasts for a long time. That's why I always recommend treating even the mildest of rashes. The box on the next page reviews the ways to manage acne-like rash.

In most cases, acne-like rashes do not leave scars, but people with light skin may be left with spots that have a reddish color, whereas darker-skinned people may have dark marks that can remain for a long time. Dermatologists call these "post-inflammatory chang-

Rash: A Step-by-Step Guide to Treatment

Severity	Treatment
Grade 1 (mild)	▪ Anti-cancer treatment can be continued at the same dose/frequency ▪ Topical corticosteroid (hydrocortisone 2.5%, triamcinolone 0.1%) **AND** Topical antibiotic (clindamycin 1–2%, erythromycin 1–2%, metronidazole 1%) twice daily ▪ Reassess in 2 weeks; if it worsens or does not improve, proceed to the next step
Grade 2 (moderate)	▪ Continue anti-cancer treatment at current dose ▪ Topical corticosteroid (hydrocortisone 2.5%, triamcinolone 0.1%) **AND** Oral antibiotic or corticosteroid for 2 to 6 weeks ▪ Reassess in 2 weeks; if it worsens or does not improve, proceed to the next step
Grade 3 (severe)	▪ Anti-cancer treatments usually interrupted or decreased by oncologist; consider testing for a skin infection ▪ Topical corticosteroid (hydrocortisone 2.5%, triamcinolone 0.1%) **AND** Oral antibiotic or corticosteroid for 2 to 6 weeks ▪ Reassess in 2 weeks; if it worsens or does not improve, oncologist may change or decrease anti-cancer treatment

es." They represent normal healing mechanisms of the skin after it has been inflamed. Rash prevention and treatment are important so these long-lasting changes can be avoided.

Chemotherapies such as taxanes (docetaxel and paclitaxel) and cyclophosphamide can also cause itchy acne-like rashes on the upper body and scalp. Corticosteroids (dexamethasone, prednisone) may cause this type of rash as well, mostly on the chest and back. Acne-like rash from corticosteroids is so common that it even has a self-explanatory name: "steroid acne."

The most effective way to treat acne-like rashes is to prevent them. Rashes from targeted therapies such as cetuximab, erlotinib, gefitinib, panitumumab, and vandetanib are usually prevented by using topical corticosteroids and oral antibiotics twice a day. Remember, there are antibiotic and corticosteroid formulations for easier scalp application: solutions, foams, and shampoos. I recommend this treatment for the first six weeks when someone starts one of the medications most often responsible (cetuximab, erlotinib, panitumumab). After that, use of the cream and antibiotic will depend on whether there is still a rash or symptoms present. This preventive treatment can reduce moderate and severe acne-like rashes from targeted therapies by more than 50 percent.

Red Rash in the Armpit and Groin

The medical term for the armpits, the area under the breasts, and groin are the intertriginous areas. These areas have special characteristics: they contain a high concentration of sweat glands, the skin always touches or rubs together, and normally there are a high number of bacteria. For unknown reasons, some medications, such as doxorubicin, are known to cause rashes in these areas. After two to four cycles of chemotherapy, redness first appears, then pain and peeling, sometimes followed by blisters. Other areas that are subject to friction or pressure, such as under a bra or belt, can also be affected.

Medications That May Cause
Armpit and Groin Rash

Doxorubicin	Sunitinib

To Treat Armpit and Groin Rashes, Use...

- Topical (hydrocortisone, triamcinolone) or oral (dexamethasone, prednisone) corticosteroids
- Topical antibiotics (mupirocin, silver sulfadiazine)
- Topical barrier creams or ointments with zinc (Desitin Maximum Strength, A+D Original Ointment, Balmex Diaper Rash Cream)

DID YOU KNOW?

Up to 32 percent of oncologists will have to stop certain anti-cancer medications because of rash, so preventing and treating rashes whenever possible are very important.

Treatments consist of topical or oral corticosteroids and antibiotics. It is easy for infections to occur in these areas of the body, so if there are any signs of infection (foul smell, discharge, intense pain, raw open skin), your doctor may obtain a culture of the skin and prescribe an antibiotic. If doxorubicin is being used, it may be necessary to reduce the dose so the skin can adjust to the injury and the treatment for the rash can take effect. As with many other chemotherapy rashes, with proper treatment, the rash tends to improve over time.

Although not as common, the targeted therapy sunitinib has been reported to cause a painful rash around the anal area and also on the scrotum in men.

Hives (or Welts) Anywhere on the Body

Hives consist of pale red, raised, itchy bumps (known as urticaria). They may be signs of an allergy to any type of medication. In most cases, hives can be treated so that anti-cancer chemotherapy or targeted therapies can continue. Hives usually appear a few minutes or hours after the offending medication is given and can appear anywhere on the body. The hives may be scattered over the body or merge together and usually are associated with burning or itching. After they heal, hives usually don't leave scars or any discoloration. Most of the time, each individual hive will last less than one day. It is important to keep track of how long each spot lasts—if more than one to two days, a dermatologist may need to do a skin biopsy to rule out a more serious type of skin disease.

Anti-cancer Medications That May Cause Hives

Alemtuzumab	Etoposide
Arsenic trioxide	Filgrastim
Asparaginase	Idarubicin
Bleomycin	Imatinib
Busulfan	Interferon
Cladribine	Interleukin
Cytarabine	Mechlorethamine
Dacarbazine	Methotrexate
Dasatinib	Mitoxantrone
Daunorubicin	Octreotide
Doxorubicin	Procarbazine
Epoetin alfa	Rituximab
Estramustine	Sorafenib

In some cases, hives indicate a more serious reaction, such as when associated with difficulty breathing. When this happens, welts develop deep in the skin and appear on the lips, eyes, or throat—a condition called angioedema. When associated with shortness of breath, fainting, and low blood pressure, the result is anaphylaxis, a life-threatening whole-body reaction. Although this serious reaction is rare, anaphylaxis is usually caused by antibiotics, aspirin, anti-seizure or pain medicines, as well as medications listed in the box on page 12, "Medicines That Can Cause Rash." It's important to tell your doctor about any other medicines, vitamins, or supplements that you may be taking in addition to chemotherapy or targeted therapy.

Surprisingly, hives can also be caused by skin contact with water, heat, cold, sunlight, pressure, or even scratching. Hives are very common in the general popu-

To Treat Hives and Welts, Use...

- Topical (fluocinonide, triamcinolone) or oral corticosteroids (dexamethasone, prednisone)
- Oral antihistamines (cetirizine, diphenhydramine, fexofenadine, hydroxyzine, loratadine)
- UV light therapy (phototherapy) at a dermatologist's office

DID YOU KNOW?

If during your appointment you have no visible hives, a test called dermatographism helps bring them out: by scratching your skin with the tip of a blunt object, a hive will come up within minutes.

lation, with about 25 percent of people developing them at some point in their lives, and almost always the cause is never known. So just because someone has hives during cancer treatment, it doesn't mean that the anti-cancer medication is causing them. Most of the time, hives are successfully treated, and no cause is found. The box above reviews the ways to manage hives and welts.

Leg Swelling or Redness

Although there are many causes for thickening and swelling of the skin of the legs (especially the shins), certain anti-cancer medications can make this happen very quickly, resulting in pain , infections, and difficulty walking. Many conditions that are already present in people living with cancer—ranging from heart disease, poor nutrition, kidney problems, low thyroid hormone, blood clots, obesity, and liver disease—can all result in some degree of leg swelling. Previous surgery or radiation therapy in the genitals, abdomen, or groin can result in swelling due to impaired draining of fluid from the skin, resulting in a condition known as lymphedema.

When doctors examine legs that are swollen, they look at the amount of swelling, whether both sides are equally large, the skin can be pinched or it dimples or hurts when pressed, and there are any open skin areas. They check the feet (athlete's foot and fungal toenail infection heighten the risk of a skin infection called cellulitis) and the groin (for enlarged lymph nodes). Tests for swollen legs may include a lymphoscintigraphy, CT or MRI, or an ultrasound. Large, bulging leg veins

Medications That May Cause Leg Swelling and Rash

Alemtuzumab	Gemcitabine	Pemetrexed
Anastrozole	Ibritumomab	Pregabalin
Bexarotene	Imatinib	Raloxifene
Corticosteroids	Interleukin-2	Rituximab
Dasatinib	L-Asparaginase	Sunitinib
Docetaxel	Lenalidomide	Tositumomab
Exemestane	Leuprolide	Trastuzumab
Fulvestrant	Nilotinib	Vorinostat
Gabapentin	Paclitaxel	

(called varices) are found in 25 percent of people, and when they hurt or have impaired blood flow, they need to be evaluated by a vascular surgeon.

Swollen legs are not just an appearance problem, as they are more prone to developing skin infections, which appear as a painful red swelling of the skin, requiring antibiotics taken as pills or through a vein. Also, swollen legs may indicate the presence of blood clots, which need to be treated with blood thinners. In either case, treatments are available, but as always, prevention is most important. Regardless of the underlying condition, certain medications used by oncologists can result in more swelling of the legs, such as the targeted therapies dasatinib, imatinib, and nilotinib or the conventional chemotherapies docetaxel, gemcitabine, paclitaxel, and pemetrexed.

In most cases, leg swelling caused by these medications can be managed so that treatment may continue. Lifestyle modifications, compression methods, keeping the legs elevated when resting, and regular exercise are all good ways to keep the swelling under control. Massage therapy by a lymphedema therapist is also an effective way to decrease the swelling and increase mobility and function of the legs.

DID YOU KNOW?

Swollen legs are very common and for many people they do not pose a problem, but they should be treated in people who are receiving medications known to cause leg swelling or when there is pain, itching, infections, or skin breakdown.

To Treat Swollen or Red Legs...

- Change lifestyle habits: Avoid prolonged standing, increase exercise, improve heart health, and control body weight
- Elevate the legs
- Wear compression stockings
- Treat large leg veins with lasers or surgery
- Get lymphedema therapy (manual lymphatic compression)
- Use topical or oral antibiotics if an infection is suspected
- Use topical corticosteroids if skin inflammation or itching from fluid backup is seen and systemic corticosteroids (dexamethasone, prednisone), especially when swelling is due to gemcitabine or pemetrexed

Rash With Painful Blisters on the Skin and Mucosae

The most serious type of rash caused by a medication consists of blisters forming all over the body, including the skin, eyes, mouth, and genitals. This rash is extremely rare but needs to be treated swiftly with intravenous medications given in the hospital, possibly in a special area dedicated to burn victims. A blister forms when water is trapped between two layers of skin. There are many causes of blisters: infections, friction, and (rarely) medicines. Blisters fill with fluid at first and then become loose before breaking open. When they rupture, the skin underneath is moist and usually painful before it dries up and crusts over. Pressing on a fluid-filled blister or scratching the skin next to a blister will extend the blister and make it larger.

When a blistering rash is caused by medication, it can involve the skin as well as the mouth, eyes, vagina, penis, or anus (the so-called mucosae). It may not be noticeable in these areas because it ruptures easily, especially in the mouth, so it appears as a painful sore. When blisters occur in the mouth, they can make it difficult to eat or drink. These severe skin reactions have the unmemorable names of Stevens–Johnson syndrome (SJS) and toxic epidermal necrolysis (TEN) and are very rare (appearing in three people out of every million), but they require urgent medical attention.

Red, Swollen Rash at the Injection SIte

In less than six percent of people receiving intravenous treatments, some amount of chemotherapy may leak into the skin. This is called an extravasation (another word for outside the blood vessel, or vein). It becomes a problem because the anti-cancer treatment can damage and inflame the skin and tissues around the leak. Rash associated with leaking chemotherapy is unpredictable and may occur at any time during the infusion.

Extravasations are less common when chemotherapy is given through a catheter or a port than when given in a vein of the arm or hand. People at higher risk for chemotherapy leaks are those with small, fragile veins; those who have frequent intravenous treatments; those with lymphedema in the arm; those who are obese or have neurologic conditions; and those who have had previous radiation therapy in the area being injected. Other factors that may increase risk include a large amount or high concentration of chemotherapy, allergy to the medication, and the blistering properties of the chemotherapy. Obviously, incorrect use of devices for the infusion and insufficient training of the personnel administering the chemotherapy will also raise the risk. It is not a life-threatening problem, so after an extravastion, chemotherapy is given through another site, either through a port, catheter, or on another side of the body, for example.

Leaks from different chemotherapies will cause distinct findings: mechlorethamine leads to inflammation of the vein, immediate pain, and poorly healing areas; oxaliplatin results in redness and swelling, then pain and ulcers; vinblastine, vincristine, and vinorelbine cause painful ulcers and numbness; pain from doxorubicin is immediate and irritation can last for months; and mitomycin C leaks can take months to show up. When chemotherapy leaks from a vein, symp-

> **DID YOU KNOW?**
>
> Approximately 8 percent of people living with cancer visit a dermatologist for a rash caused by chemotherapy or targeted therapies.

Plugging at Chemotherapy Leaks

The following are ways to treat some of the symptoms and signs of a chemotherapy leak (extravasation).

Symptoms/Signs	Treatment

Redness, swelling	- Rest and elevation of affected area
	- Local cooling or warming for 30 minutes at least four times a day
	  - Cool compresses for doxorubicin leaks
	  - Warm compresses for vinblastine, vincristine, vinorelbine leaks
	- Injected or topical antidotes
	  - Dexrazoxane antidote for daunorubicin, doxorubicin, epirubicin
	  - Topical DMSO for daunorubicin, doxorubicin, epirubicin, mitomycin C
	  - Sodium thiosulfate for mechlorethamine
	- Topical corticosteroids (hydrocortisone, triamcinolone)

Painful skin	Pain medications topically (pramoxine, lidocaine) or orally (ibuprofen, naproxen, hydrocodone, codeine, hydromorphone)
Skin breakdown, sores, or blisters	Topical antibiotics (mupirocin, Polysporin, silver sulfadiazine)
Large ulcers	Plastic surgery
Hardened skin	- Topical corticosteroids (fluocinonide, clobetasol) - Physical therapy
Skin discoloration	Bleaching creams, laser treatments
Large ulcers	Plastic surgery

toms appear within days and include swelling, pain, warmth, discomfort, and redness, followed weeks or months later by hardening and dark discoloration on the skin. Another possible complication is the formation of clots in the vein. With certain chemotherapies known as vesicants, a blister can form in the affected area up to several days after the leak. Blisters may then result in ulcers (or open areas on the skin), which take a long time to heal and may leave scars or skin discoloration.

When a chemotherapy leak is suspected, the infusion must be stopped immediately and the arm elevated above the level of the chest. Intermittent cool or warm packs (depending on the chemotherapy) are usually recommended. For specific recommendations, see the table on the previous page. Another good practice is to mark the area of skin where the leak occurred, in case additional treatment is needed, and to follow the extent of the reaction. Depending on which chemotherapy leaked, a specific type of treatment will then be given. Most oncology offices have a well-established system to deal with chemotherapy leaks. In some cases, a plastic surgeon may need to treat the site of extravasation if it is causing pain or affecting the function of that body part.

Skin Color Changes

The skin gets its color from pigments, or chemicals known as melanin. Some people produce more melanin, resulting in darker skin. Melanin protects the skin against the sun, and both sun exposure and skin inflammation will stimulate melanin production. Because people with olive or dark skin are more susceptible to more darkening, great care must be taken to prevent sun exposure and rashes during chemotherapy.

Darkening of the skin can also appear after chemotherapy. Dark areas on the face, mouth, lips, hands, and feet can gradually occur and last for a long time, if left untreated. Most of the time, dark areas are treatable, with bleaching creams or lasers administered by a dermatologist or plastic surgeon.

Some anti-cancer medications can stop the formation of skin pigment, causing skin lightening. The hair, including the eyebrows and eyelashes and even body

DID YOU KNOW?

Leakage of chemotherapy can leave the surrounding skin very hard, which may limit the ability to use that body part. Physical or occupational therapy are good ways to restore function in this situation.

Medications That May Cause Changes in Skin/Hair Color

Whitening of Skin/Hair	Darkening of Skin/Hair
Dasatinib	Bleomycin
Imatinib	Busulfan
Imiquimod	Capecitabine
Interferon	Cetuximab
Ipilimumab	Cyclophosphamide
Nilotinib	Docetaxel
Pazopanib	Doxorubicin
Sunitinib	Erlotinib
	Fluorouracil
	Gefitinib
	Paclitaxel
	Panitumumab
	Vandetanib

hair, may become gray or white. If the medication is stopped, the normal color will return. When skin gets lighter with any of these medications, it will also become more sensitive to the sun. So it's very important to be careful with sun exposure.

Anti-cancer medicines are not the only ones to cause color changes: drugs used to treat high blood pressure (diltiazem), pain or nerve conditions (gabapentin), heart conditions (amiodarone), or seizures (lamotrigine) may also be responsible, as well as certain antibiotics (minocycline).

Another phenomenon that may result in a darker color occurs after skin has become inflamed (which occurs after a rash or when a scar forms). Patients with olive or black skin are more susceptible to this, which doctors call post-inflammatory hyperpigmentation. This change is the body's defense mechanism after the skin senses an "injury." If you have olive or

To Reduce Darkening of the Skin, Use...

- Sunscreen SPF 15 or higher
- Bleaching creams (hydroquinone 4%)
- Vitamin A creams (tretinoin)
- Acid creams (azelaic acid)
- Camouflaging cosmetics
- Laser treatments or peels by a dermatologist or plastic surgeon

To Reduce Lightening of the Skin, Use...

- UV light therapy (phototherapy) in a dermatologist's office
- Camouflaging cosmetics

To Reduce Redness of the Skin, Use...

- Oxymetazoline solution
- Camouflaging cosmetics
- Laser treatments by a dermatologist or plastic surgeon

To Reduce Purple Spots on the Skin, Use...

- Vitamin A creams (tretinoin, tazarotene)
- Laser treatments by a dermatologist or plastic surgeon
- Camouflaging cosmetics

dark skin, knowing the medications that may cause rash or acne and receiving preventive or early treatment are important ways to reduce this side effect, which can last for many months.

On the other hand, fair-skinned people will develop redness after a rash or when scars form, a condition called post-inflammatory erythema. It's always

Camouflaging Cosmetics

These foundations come in many different colors, so they can be matched to your skin tone to hide rashes, blemishes, or discoloration:

- CoverFX
- AmazingCosmetics AmazingConcealer

Q My treatment for prostate cancer includes chemotherapy and corticosteroids. I'm getting these purple spots on the back of my arms that last for a long time. What are they, and is there anything I can do about them?

A Purple spots (called purpura by doctors) appear when small blood vessels under the skin break, releasing red blood cells (similar to what happens in bruises). These damaged blood cells lose oxygen and become purple. Age, sun exposure, and corticosteroids all cause thinning and weakening of the skin and its tiny blood vessels, especially on the arms, chest, and legs. Using vitamin A creams (tretinoin, tazarotene) daily, followed by a moisturizer, will help make skin stronger and prevent purple spots.

DID YOU KNOW?

If used properly, camouflaging cosmetics can conceal most skin discolorations. Using these products will not make discoloration worse.

important to rule out other causes of redness, especially on the face, such as rosacea or hot flashes. Other than camouflaging makeup, using a solution of oxymetazoline (normally used for red eyes) will shrink the tiny blood vessels temporarily. For a more permanent improvement, laser treatments performed by a dermatologist or plastic surgeon are the best choice.

Redness, Blisters, Pain in the Palms and Soles, or Hand-Foot Syndrome

A common skin reaction to anti-cancer treatments is hand-foot syndrome (HFS), which affects the palms of the hands and, more commonly, the soles of the feet. There are several reasons why these areas of the body are affected: they have more blood flow, so more of the medication reaches these areas; they are exposed to friction and trauma every day, which may cause some of the anti-cancer medicine to leak from blood vessels and cause tissue damage. Also, skin grows faster in the palms and soles than in other parts of the body, so it is more susceptible to the effects of chemotherapy. Tingling, burning, redness, blistering, tightness, swelling, numbness, and pain of the hands and/or feet are all symptoms of HFS.

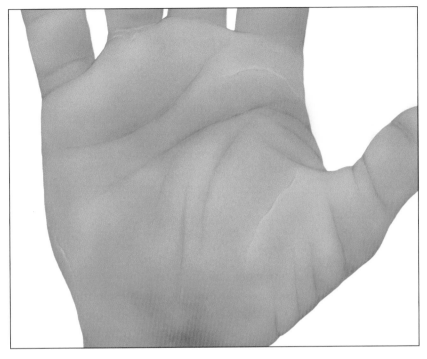

HAND-FOOT SYNDROME
Anti-cancer medicines leaking from the blood vessels or damaging the palms of the hand and soles of the feet may lead to redness, tenderness, blisters, thickening, and peeling.

Some patients are more affected in their hands, whereas most have problems in their feet. Most cases of HFS are mild and do not interfere with daily activities. However, more severe cases of HFS can affect a person's quality of life by making it difficult to walk or button clothes or handle objects. In some cases, the swelling or blisters cause the fingernails and toenails to lift and become loose and painful.

Hand-foot syndrome often begins with a sensation of tightness and pain in the hands or feet as early as two to four weeks after starting treatment. So it is especially important within the first two months of treatment to reduce vigorous activity with the hands or feet. When HFS appears, it depends on the chemotherapy or targeted therapy used. Some medications cause HFS within

Medications That May Cause Hand-Foot Syndrome

Within Two Months of Treatment	After Two Months of Treatment
Axitinib	Capecitabine
Pazopanib	Cytarabine
Sorafenib	Doxorubicin
Sunitinib	Floxuridine
	Fluorouracil
	Idarubicin
	Mitoxantrone
	Vemurafenib

the first few weeks, and others cause HFS after two or more months. Some studies have shown that 25 to 50 percent of patients treated with doxorubicin for breast or ovarian cancer experienced HFS, although fewer than half of these patients were severely affected.

Pain control is the most important aspect of treatment of HFS, so your doctor may recommend oral non-steroidal anti-inflammatories, corticosteroids, or opioids. Topical medicines also can be used, including corticosteroids, anesthetics, or moisturizing exfoliants.

To Treat Hand-Foot Syndrome...

- For thickened or callused areas: topical moisturizers that exfoliate (creams containing urea, ammonium lactate, or salicylic acid)
- For red or painful areas: topical corticosteroids (clobetasol, fluocinonide, or halobetasol)
- For pain from liposomal doxorubicin: oral corticosteroids (dexamethasone)
- For symptoms from capecitabine: oral non-steroidal anti-inflammatories (celecoxib, ibuprofen, naproxen)
- For pain from any chemotherapy: topical anesthetics (benzocaine, lidocaine), oral opioids (codeine, hydrocodone, hydromorphone)

To Reduce the Risk of Hand-Foot Syndrome...

During the first month, avoid excessive pressure or friction on the hands and feet. Avoid hot baths or showers.

Wear protective gloves and socks
- Cotton gloves (Walgreens 100% Cotton Gloves, Cara Cotton Gloves) during activities using the hands
- Vinyl gloves when washing dishes
- Thick (Thorlos) or toe-protecting socks (Injinji, Happy Feet Original Foot Alignment Socks, SmartWool) when walking
- Gel-lined gloves and socks at night after applying creams or ointments (Women's Terry, Bliss, XpresSpa)

Care for blisters
- Do not break them open
- Apply Dr. Scholl's Blister Treatment Cushions

Remove thick, callused areas with files or topical medications
- Peel the thick skin: Derma-Seta Spa Kit, Sof Feet Callus Reducer, PedEgg, Kmart Pedi Spin, Dr. Scholl's Callus Reducer
- Soften the areas: Dr. Scholl's Liquid Corn & Callus Remover, Walgreens Medicated Callus Removers Kit, Callus Care Complete Callus Care with Pumice Stone

Always wear soft padded footwear, such as the following:
- Slippers: Crocs footwear, Tempur-Pedic
- Shoes: Crocs footwear, UGG, Mephisto, Merrell, Orthaheel, Arcopedico, Orthofeet Stretchable

Use friction or pressure reducing products
- Dr. Scholl's Rub Relief Stick and Strips
- Use calfskin (Dr. Scholl's Moleskin or Molefoam Padding) in areas of pressure
- Use insoles: New Balance Pressure Relief, Shock Doctor Ultra, ArchCrafters Custom Fit

Use cushions in affected areas
- Sides of foot: Dr. Scholl's Corn Cushions, FootSmart Gel/Felt Cushions, FootSmart Silicone Bunionette Shield, FootSmart Metatarsal Sleeve
- Toes: FootSmart Digi-Cushion, MenthoGel Toe Protector Tubes, FootSmart Gel Toe Cap, FootSmart Toe Socks, FootSmart U-shaped Gel Toe Separators
- Ball of the foot: FootSmart Gel Ball-of-Foot Cushion, FootSmart Silicone Plantar Cushion with Gel
- Heel: Dr. Scholl's P.R.O. inserts for Heel, Dr. Scholl's Massaging Gel Heel Cups

Your oncologist may decide to temporarily stop or reduce the dose of the anti-cancer medication triggering HFS if the pain is limiting your ability to walk or care for yourself. Once HFS has improved, the medication can be started, sometimes at a lower dose to prevent a recurrence of HFS.

Skin Bumps and Growths

One of the most peculiar side effects from the new targeted therapies is the formation of tiny bumps on the skin that look like warts and may make the skin feel sandpaper-like. The medications that cause this phenomenon are sorafenib and vemurafenib. In most cases, these growths occur within the first two to three months of therapy, and up to 20 percent of people may develop them. They can appear anywhere on the body, but most frequently they appear on the face, neck, back, and arms. In most cases, they are just a cosmetic issue, although they can become a nuisance, as they can bleed or get caught in clothes. In less that five percent of people on vemurafenib, skin cancers may also develop. Fortunately, they are not nearly as dangerous as melanoma, and can be easily treated by a dermatologist through a small procedure done in the office.

THINGS TO REMEMBER

- A rash is not a specific diagnosis but rather a term referring to many different clinical presentations or diseases that are frequently caused by medications.

- Let your doctor or nurse know if you experience a rash during your cancer treatment, especially if you are having signs of an infection, allergic reaction, or blisters.

- Many anti-cancer medications, but also antibiotics, anti-seizure, and anti-inflammatory medicines, can cause rashes.

- Hand-foot syndrome is one of the most common rashes to anti-cancer medications. Gentle care and topical and oral medications will usually address the most important symptom: pain.

- Rashes caused by targeted therapies (such as bortezomib, cetuximab, erlotinib, and panitumumab) may be a sign that the treatment is working. Treating the rash, however, will not affect the effectiveness of the medication.

- There are many ways to treat or prevent most rashes; in most cases, rashes should not interfere with continued cancer treatment.

- Although most rashes are not related to infections, the skin where they appear may become infected, requiring topical or oral antibiotics.

- Some anticancer medications (sorafenib and vemurafenib) may cause skin bumps and growths, which can be treated with local measures so that treatment may continue.

- When rashes are severe or intolerable, your oncologist may decide to hold or decrease the anti-cancer medication. Treating the rash should continue to prevent a recurrence of symptoms.

CHAPTER 3

Taking Care of Dry Skin

D ry skin (called "xerosis" by doctors) can feel scaly, tight, itchy, and also painful. It may even become red and swollen. But dry skin is not just one more annoying cosmetic problem. Left untreated, dry skin can lead to itching and a loss of fluid in the body (because the skin loses its ability to retain water). Dry skin may also lead to infections (from scratching or cracks, both of which allow infection-causing bacteria or viruses to enter the body). Dry skin can also result in allergies (eczema), folliculitis (an infection of the hair follicles), and cellulitis (a potentially serious bacterial infection of the skin's underlying tissues). When the skin dries, the discomfort and itch can reduce the quality of life, and the ability to sleep may be affected. It may also be difficult to work or play when the skin on the hands or feet is very dry.

DID YOU KNOW?

People living with cancer report that dry skin is one of the most important and unexpected side effects of treatment.

How Doctors Grade Dry Skin

Your doctor or nurse will determine what kind of moisturizer and/or topical medications you may need based on the severity of the dryness. Dry skin is measured primarily by its extent, appearance, and associated symptoms. See the table on the next page, and you will be able to grade your dryness. Another factor that is taken into consideration is how much of your skin is affected and whether the dryness will improve with over-the-counter creams or ointments.

Grading Dry Skin

Severity	Characteristics
Mild	Dryness covering less than 10 percent of the surface of the body, with no redness, irritation, or itching
Moderate	Dryness covering between 10 percent and 30 percent of the surface of the body, with redness, irritation, or itching, which affects the ability to do daily activities such as preparing meals, shopping, using the telephone, handling money, etc.
Severe	Dryness covering more than 30 percent of the surface of the body, with redness, irritation, or itching, which can affect the ability to do activities such as bathing, dressing and undressing, eating, using the toilet, or taking medications.

DID YOU KNOW?

There are more than 200 known causes of dry skin, and there are 32 different types of anti-cancer treatments known to cause dry skin.

In this chapter, you'll learn more about what causes dry skin, how to prevent and treat it, and the best ways to moisturize your skin.

Causes of Dry Skin

The skin is continually renewing itself by growing new cells quickly in its deep layers and sloughing off old cells at the surface. This surface layer is filled with proteins and oily chemicals, which enable skin to retain water inside the body. That's vital for the body in general, and the skin in particular, since most of its moisture comes from water and nutrients carried by underlying blood vessels.

Although skin is often driest on the lips, hands, feet, and lower legs, this pattern varies from person to person. The lower legs have few oil glands and less blood flow. The hands are constantly being washed or in contact with cleaning products, which is why they dry out so easily. Lips have no oil glands; unlike the skin on the rest of the body, lip tissue has no thick, protective outer layer. Also, the lips are continually moistened by saliva and then dried by breathing. Hands (from washing) and feet (from sweating) tend to dry out as well. Thicker skin on the elbows and knees has trouble retaining water, and its constant exposure to friction is also drying.

Dry skin is caused or made more severe by many factors:

- Age (about 75 percent of people over age 75 have dry skin)
- Genetics (some people are predisposed to dry skin)
- Medical issues (eczema, diabetes, thyroid deficiency; kidney or liver diseases; autoimmmune diseases such as lupus; HIV and HTLV-2 infection; allergies; or nutritional deficiencies)
- Perfume and scented products, such as soaps, detergents, gels, and lotions
- Frequent washing with soap or hot water
- Environmental conditions (cold temperatures, sun exposure, air conditioners, and heaters)
- Smoking
- How much time a person spends outdoors (especially in sunny or cold conditions) and whether he or she lives at a high altitude or away from a lake or ocean; places with a drier climate
- Medications and treatments such as anti-estrogen and lipid-lowering medicines, chemotherapies, targeted therapies, radiation therapy, and stem cell or bone marrow transplants
- Hodgkin lymphoma, non-Hodgkin lymphoma

Preventing and Treating Dry Skin

To protect your skin from drying out, there are a number of things you can control in your environment, such as keeping the air in your home moist by lowering the heat or using a warm-mist humidifier. Also, avoiding long showers or baths and hot water is key. Perfumed or scented soaps or gels, sun exposure, and the use of loofahs or scrubs during the shower

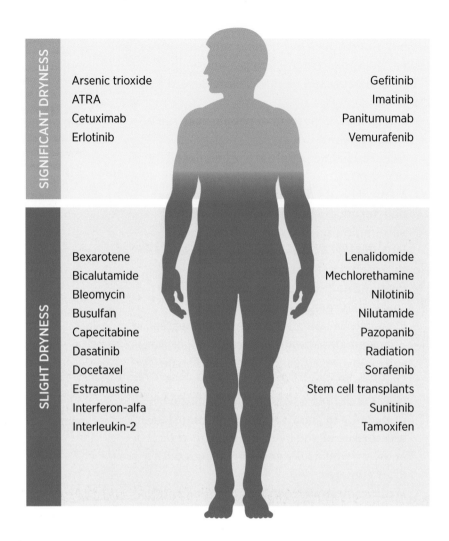

SIGNIFICANT DRYNESS

Arsenic trioxide
ATRA
Cetuximab
Erlotinib

Gefitinib
Imatinib
Panitumumab
Vemurafenib

SLIGHT DRYNESS

Bexarotene
Bicalutamide
Bleomycin
Busulfan
Capecitabine
Dasatinib
Docetaxel
Estramustine
Interferon-alfa
Interleukin-2

Lenalidomide
Mechlorethamine
Nilotinib
Nilutamide
Pazopanib
Radiation
Sorafenib
Stem cell transplants
Sunitinib
Tamoxifen

ANTI-CANCER TREATMENTS THAT MAY DRY OUT YOUR SKIN
The dryness caused by these medications may vary in severity and appear in different locations on the body.

should also be avoided. However, it's important to follow proper hygiene, as cancer treatment can increase your susceptibility to infections. Always wash your hands or use an antibacterial hand sanitizer before applying skin care products, and close lids of products tightly. Never share skin care products, and always replace them according to the manufacturer's recommendations or expiration dates.

Q I was told to apply a lot of lotion and drink a lot of water to prevent skin dryness. Will this be enough?

A Drinking at least eight glasses of water a day may certainly be important for overall health but will not be sufficient to keep your skin moisturized. You also need to reduce your skin's exposure to water, soaps, and fragrances and maintain a humid environment at home. In addition, frequent use (at least two times a day and even more frequently if receiving a chemotherapy that causes skin dryness) of thick moisturizers is always better, so use ointments or creams over lotions.

Q What is the best way to add humidity to the dry air in my home?

A A number of techniques can help: place pans of water near heating vents, hang damp laundry inside on racks, leave the bathroom door open after a warm shower, avoid using the "high" setting on heating or air-conditioning. Humidifiers are an efficient way to add moisture to the air. There are several types: warm-mist humidifiers (also called steam or evaporative) are preferable to cool-mist humidifiers (also called ultrasonic or impeller). The warm-mist machines create fewer pollutants, so they may be a better choice for people living with cancer. All humidifiers must be carefully cleaned and maintained to avoid a buildup of germs, which could result in infections.

Using Moisturizers

Moisturizers create a barrier on the skin that prevents water from escaping. This allows dry skin to heal. The best way to use moisturizers is to apply them after bathing or showering. Pat the skin dry and then apply the moisturizer. Re-apply at night before going to bed. Store shelves are filled with various types of moisturizers: ointments, creams, lotions. Many brands will have one or several of each, so read the label carefully to make sure you are getting the recommended one. Some contain sunscreen, and others contain an exfoliant to remove flaky skin. Which is the best one for you?

Ointments are 80 percent oil and 20 percent water. They're very thick and may be difficult to spread over large areas of the body. Ointments provide the

DID YOU KNOW?

The outermost layer of skin is 15 percent to 20 percent water; once it falls below 10 percent, flakes or scales appear—typical signs of dry skin.

Dehydration and Your Dry Skin

Everything in your body contains fluid (water). The human body must have between 55 percent and 75 percent water. Reduced fluid in the body can change how a person feels. Fluid balance means that the body's fluids are properly regulated and in the right places: too much water in the body, and swelling occurs; not enough water in the body–and dehydration sets in. We lose about 12 cups of water a day, including one cup from the soles of our feet.

The signs and symptoms of dehydration include:

- Dry mouth and/or excessive thirst
- Dizziness, weakness, and constipation
- Difficulty swallowing dry food
- Dry or sticky mouth which make it difficult to talk
- Dry skin that "tents" (stays up) when lightly pinched
- A swollen, cracked, or dry tongue or fingertips
- Little or no urine

Be sure to tell your doctor or nurse if you believe you are dehydrated. Your health care team may give you fluids intravenously.

best moisturization, but they look and feel greasy, so some people don't find them acceptable. Examples of ointments are petroleum jelly (Vaseline), Lubriderm Intense Skin Repair Ointment, and Vaniply Ointment.

Creams are 50 percent oil and 50 percent water. They're less thick and easier to spread than ointments.

I am starting chemotherapy soon. I know my skin is dry, but it doesn't really affect me. So why should I bother to apply moisturizers?

Dry skin is not just a matter of appearance. In fact, it's important to keep skin well moisturized as part of overall health. That's because dryness may progress to itching and scratching, which can lead to infections as well as a greater loss of water from the body. Most anti-cancer treatments will make skin drier, so it is important to prevent potential complications by keeping skin well moisturized.

Q I'm worried about getting an infection during my treatment, so I wash my hands many times a day. Will this make the dryness on my hands worse? If so, what can I do to prevent infections?

A Washing hands with antibacterial or fragranced soaps and hot water will make your skin even drier. Be sure to use a gentle, fragrance-free soap and lukewarm water or hand-sanitizing antibacterial gels instead. Antibacterial gels are more effective at destroying bacteria and, when combined with emollients, cause less dryness than washing with soap and water. Also be sure to moisturize your hands when you finish washing them.

Creams are usually white, are packaged in a tub or a tube, and are absorbed by the skin within 10 to 15 minutes of application. Examples of creams preferred by dermatologists include Aveeno Intense Relief Moisturizing Cream, Vanicream Skin Cream, CeraVe Moisturizing Cream, Eucerin Original Moisturizing Creme, and Cetaphil Moisturizing Cream.

DID YOU KNOW?

Dry skin usually begins in the legs and then spreads to other parts of the body. When skin becomes very dry, it can itch, which often starts at night.

Lotions are similar to creams but are even lighter and less thick. Lotions are the easiest to spread over large areas of the body and are sold in squeezable tubes or bottles with pumps. But because they are so thin, lotions may not be as effective for severely dry or sensitive skin. If you do use a lotion, look at the list of ingredients to make sure it does not contain alcohol, which can irritate the skin. Recommended lotions are Aveeno Skin Relief Moisturizing Lotion Fragrance Free, Cetaphil Moisturizing Lotion, CeraVe Moisturizing Lotion, Lubriderm Daily Moisture Lotion Fragrance-Free, and Vanicream Lite Lotion.

Different moisturizers have different functions.

Emollients, such as lanolin, mineral oil, and petroleum jelly (Vaseline), fill in the spaces between the cells in the skin, helping replace oils and thus smoothing and lubricating rough skin. Petroleum jelly and mineral oil are safe to be used as moisturizers. Emollients are either oil-based (a small amount of water is dissolved in oil) or

Q I'm receiving a treatment for lung cancer that makes my skin very dry, especially my hands. These painful cracks that look like paper cuts have formed in my fingers and heels. Help!

A In the hands and heels, dry skin may manifest itself as painful cracks, or "fissures." It can be made worse by repeated washing. Frequent use of heavy moisturizers containing zinc oxide such as Desitin Maximum Strength, A+D Original Ointment, Balmex Diaper Rash Cream with ActivGuard or O'Keeffe's Working Hands Creme is recommended. Use gloves and socks lined with gel at night to trap the moisturizers (Women's Terry Gel-Lined, Bliss, XpresSpa Hydrating Gel Gloves and Socks).

DID YOU KNOW?

Dry skin is not caused by not drinking sufficient amounts of water. It is caused because cells in the outer layer of the skin become dehydrated, disorganized and frayed, resulting in a scaly, flaky texture.

water-based (they primarily contain water and have a light, non-greasy feel). It's important to note that about three percent of people are allergic to lanolin, an ingredient in some emollients such as Aquaphor, which comes from the wool wax of sheep. If you're not sure whether you are allergic to lanolin, try a small amount on a small area of skin on your forearm or behind your ear (leaving it covered with a bandage for one to two days before removing it), to find out whether you have any reaction to it (such as redness, swelling, or itching).

Exfoliants, such as ammonium lactate (AmLactin cream, Lac-Hydrin 12% cream), salicylic acid (6% cream), and urea (Nutraplus Therapeutic Cream, Udderly Smooth Extra Care, and Hydro 40 Foam, Carmol

Q Is there anything else I can use to cover or heal these painful cracks in my fingertips or heels?

A Use barriers to keep germs out and moisture in. Liquid bandages are a useful mixture of chemicals that form a barrier when applied. Good examples are Band-Aid Liquid Bandage or New-Skin Antiseptic Liquid Bandage and Nexcare Skin Crack Care. You can also use fingertip bandages (these are "H" or hourglass shaped) or "cots" after applying thick creams, to retain moisture and prevent pain when using the fingers.

LOTIONS CREAMS OINTMENTS

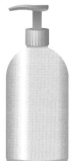 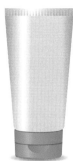 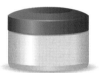

EASIEST
APPLICATION

INTERMEDIATE MOISTURE RETENTION
AND
EASE OF APPLICATION

BEST MOISTURE
RETENTION

USING MOISTURIZERS TO PREVENT AND TREAT DRY SKIN
The extent and severity of dry skin will determine what product is the best to use. Lotions are easier to apply to large areas, whereas ointments are more moisturizing. Creams are in the middle in both ease of application and ability to moisturize.

10%–40%) creams, remove inert skin cells from the top skin layer, allowing new, rejuvenated skin to surface. The newer skin now absorbs moisture more easily, so the skin feels and looks less dry. Although exfoliants can help the look of your skin, they can sting when applied and damage skin that is sensitive, dry, or red, so try them in a small spot and leave them on for 10-15 minutes before using them over a large area. Exfoliant application may also be followed by a moisturizer, to minimize irritation.

With all of these options, there are a few things to keep in mind:

- Heavier, oil-based ointments are the best to keep your skin moist.
- Moisturizers that contain sunscreen are recommended for people who spend time outdoors (See Chapter 10, "Sun Safety").

Washing and Moisturizing the Face
A good facial wash and moisturizer are important tools in skin care. The skin on your face is thinner and

> **DID YOU KNOW?**
> Dryness of the scalp and face may be dandruff, so consult a dermatologist when in doubt for the correct treatment.

Moisturizer Guide: Scalp and Face

	Scalp	Face
Dryness	• Free & Clear Shampoo and Conditioner • Aveda Scalp Remedy Dandruff Solution • Kiehl's Enriched Massage Oil for Scalp	• Aveeno Ultra-Calming Daily Moisturizer SPF 30 • Vanicream Skin Cream or Lite Lotion • Cetaphil Restoraderm Skin Restoring Moisturizer • CeraVe Facial Moisturizing Lotion PM
Dryness with flaking	• Fluocinolone scalp oil • Ciclopirox 1% shampoo	• Hydrocortisone 1% cream or ointment • Aveeno Creamy Moisturizing Oil • Eucerin Redness Relief Soothing Night Creme
Dryness with flaking and itching or redness	• Clobetasol or fluocinonide solution • Clobetasol or betamethasone foam • Clobetasol shampoo	• Hydrocortisone 2.5% or Pramosone cream • Alclometasone cream

DID YOU KNOW?

Some anti-cancer therapies can cause dry hair. Aveda Brilliant Humectant Pomade or Brilliant Emollient Finishing Gloss or Nexxus Sleekstyle Calming Smoothing Crème may be helpful.

more sensitive than elsewhere, so it's a good idea to use different products on your face than on your body. Products labeled "non-comedogenic" are preferable because they will not clog your pores. Choose a facial cleanser and moisturizer that are right for your skin type. Recommended facial cleansers include Aveeno Ultra-Calming Moisturizing Cream Cleanser, CeraVe Hydrating Cleanser, Cetaphil Daily Facial Cleanser, Eucerin Redness Relief Soothing Cleanser, and Free & Clear Liquid Cleanser. If you have sensitive skin, it's best to use products labeled hypoallergenic (less likely to cause allergies).

If you have oily skin, find a moisturizer that is light and oil-free. Keep in mind that you may need a light

Moisturizer Guide: Body and Hands/Feet

	Body	Hands and/or Feet
Dryness	▪ Dove Cream Oil Shea Butter Body Lotion ▪ Aveeno Advanced Care Moisturizing Cream and Intense Relief Repair Cream ▪ Eucerin Calming Creme Daily Moisturizer ▪ Vanicream Skin Cream ▪ Cetaphil Moisturizing Cream ▪ CeraVe Moisturizing Cream	▪ Dove Cream Oil Intensive Hand Cream ▪ Aveeno Intense Relief Hand Cream ▪ Vaniply Ointment ▪ Cetaphil Therapeutic Hand Cream ▪ CeraVe Moisturizing Cream ▪ Eucerin Original Moisturizing Creme ▪ Vaseline Healing Hand Cream
Dryness with flaking	▪ Lactic acid, ammonium lactate creams; salicylic acid (CeraVe SA Renewing Lotion) ▪ Urea (Nutraplus Therapeutic Cream, Udderly Smooth Extra Care)	▪ Urea cream (Nutraplus Therapeutic Cream, Udderly Smooth Extra Care, Carmol 10 or 40 Cream, Umecta Mousse, and Hydro 40 Foam) ▪ Salicylic acid 6% cream
Dryness with flaking and itching or redness	▪ Triamcinolone or mometasone cream	▪ Fluocinonide or betamethasone cream

lotion in the summer and a heavy cream or ointment in the winter. To get the most out of a moisturizer, use it when your skin is still damp, after patting dry with a soft towel. Because moisturizers keep moisture in, the skin needs to have some moisture in it: If the skin is too wet, the moisturizer will simply drip off; if the skin is too dry, it won't be as effective. Gently pat your face dry after washing and apply the moisturizer within 15 minutes. You should apply a facial moisturizer at least twice a day.

Q When I shower, I use an antibacterial soap, since I am worried about infections, and it also smells nice. Should I continue using this soap during my chemotherapy?

A To reduce skin dryness, it's best to avoid soaps such as Zest, Ivory, Irish Spring, Dial, Lever2000, or Coast, all of which are antibacterial and perfumed. The best choices are the soaps from Vanicream, fragrance-free Dove, Cetaphil, Aveeno, or Basis. Remember to shower with lukewarm water for just five to ten minutes and pat your skin dry. It may seem odd, but long showers and bathing dry the skin.

The skin that surrounds the eyes is somewhat different from the skin on other areas of the face. However, you can use your facial moisturizer in this area. Moisturizers specifically designed for around the eyes are usually the same products but just more expensive and in a different container.

You don't have to buy expensive facial moisturizers—just the right one for you. Facial moisturizers that are gentle include Vanicream Skin Cream or Lite Lotion, Cetaphil Restoraderm Skin Restoring Moisturizer, CeraVe Facial Moisturizing Lotion PM, and Eucerin Redness Relief Soothing Night Creme.

The Truth About Hand Sanitizers Although most people believe that alcohol-based hand sanitizers are more drying and irritating than hand washing with soap, it turns out they are less drying, especially if they contain emollients. Another benefit of hand sanitizers is their ability to destroy more than 99 percent of bacteria, viruses, and fungi on the hands. A concentration of at least 60 percent alcohol is recommended, and application should be enough to wet or cover hands completely. It should be done after preparing foods; using the bathroom; touching other people, dirty objects, or animals; and coughing or sneezing. It is also recommended that application occur before cooking, taking medicines, and touching someone who is ill or injured. Examples of alcohol-based sanitizers include Purell, Germ-X, Lysol, and

Tips for Taking Care of Dry Skin

Keep baths or showers short. If you prefer bathing, take an oatmeal bath with Aveeno Soothing Bath Treatment, Skin Relief Shower and Bath Oil, Foaming Bath, or Vanicream's RoBathol Bath Oil. Be careful when using bath oils, since they will make your tub very slippery.

Use cool or lukewarm water, not hot water.

Avoid scrubbing skin with loofahs or sponges during showers or baths, as they irritate the skin and are loaded with germs.

After showering or bathing, apply a fragrance-free hypoallergenic body moisturizer while your skin is still damp (usually within 15 minutes). Be sure to apply the moisturizer all over: arms, elbows, hands, legs, feet, abdomen, and back. Moisturizers should be applied twice a day, especially after baths or showers and on your hands every time you wash them or do any cleaning.

Avoid colognes, gels, aftershaves, and after-bath splashes that contain alcohol.

Use fragrance-free detergents such as Dreft, All Free Clear, Cheer Free & Gentle, Arm & Hammer Liquid Detergent HE Compatible, Seventh Generation Free & Clear, or Tide Free & Gentle.

Drink plenty of liquids each day (check with your doctor or nurse first about the ideal amount for you).

Protect your skin from cold, wind, and sun; avoid heat, especially dry heat.

Wear soft fabrics, such as cotton, and avoid tight clothes or underwear. Using camisoles (instead of bras) and boyshorts (instead of panties) helps minimize irritation in dry areas under and on the sides of the chest and in the groin.

Method, and these products are preferred over those containing other chemicals such as triclosan or benzalkonium chloride. Some natural products are Clean Well All Natural Hand Sanitizer, Burt's Bees Aloe & Witch Hazel Hand Sanitizer, and EO Natural Hand Sanitizer.

Moisturizing Mucosae

The tissues that cover the lips, eyes, inside of the mouth, ears, nose, and genitals are called mucosae. These tissues can also become dry with chemotherapy, radiation therapy, and after stem cell transplants.

Dry Eyes

Dry eyes are a frequent and often underrecognized symptom in people living with cancer. Dry eyes can be uncomfortable and may cause blurry vision; they may interfere with the ability to do daily activities. Chemotherapies that frequently cause dry eyes include ATRA, cetuximab, docetaxel, erlotinib, gefitinib, paclitaxel, and panitumumab. Contact lenses and other medicines that may also cause dry eyes include anti-allergy drugs (diphenhydramine [Benadryl], hydroxyzine [Atarax]).

Treatment with artificial tears (Systane Ultra High Performance Lubricant Eye Drops, GenTeal Lubricant Eye Gel or Tears Severe Dry Eye Relief, Visine Tears Lubricant Eye Drops) used up to four times a day can help. Some people need to use these medications more frequently; in such cases, it's better to use a preservative-free formula (Clear Eyes Tears Preservative Free, Tears Naturale Free). When using gel tears, it's best to apply them before going to sleep, since they can cause temporary blurry vision. An evaluation by an ophthalmologist is always advisable if you experience eye symptoms, as there may be other causes, including allergies and blockage of the ducts that carry tears. Ophthalmologists may suggest additional methods such as Thermoeyes Moisture Release Eyewear, artifical tear inserts (Lacrisert), or tear duct plugs.

When dryness occurs on the sides of the nose, it is usually dandruff. When the dryness appears in or around the nostrils it may be associated with crusting, tenderness, and occasional bleeding. This dryness occurs from inflammation of an area inside the nose by infectious bacteria, most commonly *Staphylococcus*. Chemotherapies that cause dry skin (especially cetuximab, erlotinib, gefitinib, and panitumumab) or excessive nose blowing or picking may all trigger this problem. It can be treated with topical antibiotics mupirocin (Bactroban) or Polysporin ointment twice daily for two weeks and then twice daily on the weekends, as long as symptoms last. Obtaining a bacterial culture of the nostrils is also recommended, so that the exact bacterium causing the inflammation can be identified. In addition to the topical antibiotics, using moisturizing sprays (Ayr Saline Nasal Gel, Oasis) frequently during the day is also helpful.

Dry Mouth

Dry mouth is a problem because saliva plays an important role. Too little saliva can result in cavities, yeast infections, and gum disease; changes in the ability to taste and speak; difficulty chewing and swallowing; and lack of appetite.

In addition to over-the-counter gums and liquids, artificial saliva sprays or lozenges can be used. Your doctor can also prescribe tablets that stimulate the formation of saliva, such as cevimeline (30-mg tablets three times a day) or pilocarpine (5-mg tablets three times a day). If dry mouth is aggravated by the growth of a yeast called Candida, thrush occurs. When this happens, tongue or mouth pain, along with red or whitish bumps or plaques, appears. Treatment for thrush is nystatin suspension, nystatin lozenges, or clotrimazole lozenges four times a day; miconazole (Oravig buccal) tablets may also be used daily for two weeks. Sometimes yeast infections affect the corners of the mouth, causing tenderness and irritation. This condition can be treated with the antifungal miconazole or nystatin cream or ointment two to four times a day.

Dry or chapped lips are a common complaint, especially in the winter. Allergies, infections, and chemotherapy-induced inflammation can cause painful, chapped lips; so too can many targeted therapies such as: cetuximab, erlotinib, gefitinib, panitumumab, or sorafenib. If your lips feel dry, use a heavy ointment, such as petroleum jelly (Vaseline) many times a day (up to six or more). If you have lip pain, use a topical corticosteroid, such as hydrocortisone 2.5% ointment. An evaluation by a dermatologist is important to rule out allergies or sensitivity to the sun. Your dermatol-

Dry Mouth: What Works

Method	Names	Efficacy/ Time of Effect
Gum	Biotene Dry Mouth Gum OMNI TheraGum Spry Chewing Gum XyliChew Gum Orbit Sugarfree Gum	Minimal/ brief duration
Lozenge	SalivaSure lozenges Numoisyn lozenges	Moderate/ brief duration
Disc	OraMoist Dry Mouth Disc	Minimal/ several hours
Liquids	Biotene spray Aquoral Artificial Saliva Mouth Kote Dry Mouth Spray Numoisyn Liquid	Moderate/ brief duration
Mouth hygiene	Biotene Alcohol-Free Mouthwash Biotene PBF Toothpaste Dentiva Oral Hygiene Lozenge MedActive Oral Rinse Oasis Mouthwash PreviDent 5000 Rinse and Toothpaste Sensodyne Toothpaste Sonicare Air Floss and Toothbrush	Good/ intermediate duration
Saliva stimulants	Cevimeline tablets Pilocarpine tablets	Good/ several hours

ogist may do an allergy test (called a patch test) or a swab culture of your lips to find out whether there is an infection. If there is no improvement, a biopsy of the lip may be needed. When using topical medications on the

Q My lips are very dry and chapped, so I lick them to keep them moist. Is this OK?

A No. Frequently (at least four times a day) use ointments (such as petroleum jelly [regular Vaseline or Vaseline Lip Therapy Petroleum Jelly, Advanced Formula]). Try to avoid licking them. Saliva is irritating and can make dryness worse. In cases where there is lip pain with cracking, use a topical corticosteroid (hydrocortisone 2.5% ointment) applied together with an antibacterial (Polysporin First Aid Antibiotic Ointment); up to three times a day is a useful treatment for several weeks at a time.

lips, applying a thin layer is usually enough. If a small amount gets in your mouth, it should not be a concern.

Vaginal Dryness

Vaginal dryness is very common, especially with increasing age, after menopause (either natural or induced by chemotherapy), and with certain hormonal treatments such as anastrozole, fulvestrant, leuprolide, medroxyprogesterone, octreotide, raloxifene, or tamoxifen. When vaginal dryness occurs, over-the-counter lubricants such as Astroglide Natural, K-Y Silk-E, or Replens can help. In some cases, your doctor (or your gynecologist) may prescribe vaginal estrogen creams (Premarin, Estrace), tablets (Vagifem), inserts (Lubrin), or rings (Estring). The use of vaginal estrogen should be monitored by your doctor, especially if used for a long time.

THINGS TO REMEMBER

- All anti-cancer treatments, including chemotherapy, radiation therapy, and stem cell transplants, can cause dry skin.

- Dry skin on the hands and feet that is left untreated can result in painful cracks or fissures, which may affect the ability to do daily activities.

- Water evaporating from skin will dehydrate it, so make sure to pat dry with a soft absorbent towel, after washing, showering, or bathing; apply a moisturizer within 15 minutes.

- Place a moisturizer in several places around your home, car, and office, so you always have it handy to apply several times a day.

- The tissue that covers the lips, eyes, lining of the mouth, ears, nose, and genitals is called mucosa; it can also become dry as a result of chemotherapy, radiation therapy, and stem cell transplants.

- When dry skin itches, both the dryness and the itching must be treated. Using a topical corticosteroid cream or ointment will also provide some moisturization.

- If you are using a topical medication, apply it first, and then wait until it is dry before applying a moisturizer. The skin on your face is thinner and more sensitive than skin elsewhere, so it's a good idea to use a different moisturizer on your face than on the rest of your body.

- Dryness and flaking on the scalp and face can frequently represent dandruff. Seek an evaluation by a dermatologist for appropriate treatment with corticosteroid and antifungal creams, lotions, or shampoos.

- Avoid using soaps or detergents that are antibacterial or scented, as they dry the skin. Hand washing makes skin drier as well, so be sure to use a moisturizer after you wash your hands or antibacterial hand sanitizers with emollients.

How to Stop the Itching

Itching—or pruritus, as doctors call it—is an uncomfortable skin sensation, familiar to many people living with cancer. In fact, nearly one in five people experiences severe itching during his or her lifetime—that is, a constant irritating itch, as opposed to the occasional need to scratch, which everyone has at one time or another. Itch can cause discomfort and may be frustrating to cope with. If not well managed, itch sometimes leads to difficulty sleeping, anxiety, trouble concentrating, and even depression in the most severe cases. Skin that is frequently scratched can then become infected or thick and leathery—a condition called lichenification. These patches of skin may be raw, red, or darker than the rest of the skin. Persistent scratching can also lead to permanent scars or changes in skin color.

In this chapter, you will learn about the different causes of itching; ways to prevent and treat itchy skin; and specific medications that can help, both over-the-counter and prescription. Although many cases of itchy skin go away on their own, others may require treatment, especially if caused by anti-cancer medications.

What Causes Itching?

Although the exact mechanism of itch is unknown, it is believed to be a complex process involving nerves that respond to certain chemicals released in the skin that send signals through nerves going to the brain. The triggers for the release of these chemicals in the skin include medicines (topical or oral), vibration, heat, or injuries. In these instances, itch can be treated locally (with topical medications) or systemically (with oral medicines that affect the release of chemicals in the skin or brain). Itching can also result from irritation in the nerves that run under the skin or even those located in the brain. In order to choose the right type of treatment, it's important to determine the origin of the itch.

Itch can occur as a result of various diseases, including a skin disease itself; kidney, liver, or neurologic diseases; or iron deficiency (anemia). Things that irritate the skin, such as soaps, detergents, fragrances, clothing, or anything that the skin comes in contact with can trigger or aggravate it, even with products that have been used for many years. Dry skin and even aging can lead to itch by allowing irritants to penetrate the skin more readily. With anti-cancer treatments, the skin also becomes a less effective barrier to such irritants, allowing them to cause itch.

Cancer can also cause itch for reasons that are not clear, but which may include the formation of certain pro-itch chemicals or direct effects on the function of the kidneys, liver, or nerves. When caused by cancer, itch usually appears on the legs, upper chest and back, and front of the arms. As the cancer is treated, the itch usually goes away.

A number of cancers are likely to cause itch as a symptom on different parts of the body:
- Brain tumors (on the nose)
- Leukemia (trunk and extremities)
- Lymphoma (frequently on the arms or legs and with dryness)
- Melanoma (at the site of the lesion)
- Pancreatic cancer (trunk and extremities)
- Lung cancer (trunk and extremities)
- Breast cancer (during radiation or on areas of skin metastases)
- Stomach cancer (trunk and extremities)
- Prostate cancer (on the scrotum)

- Cervical cancer (vagina)
- Rectal cancer (anus)
- Blood cell cancers such as mastocytosis, polycythemia vera, myelodysplastic syndromes (on the trunk and extremities)

Itch can also occur as a result of cancer treatments and may be associated with a rash, hives, or dry skin. Sometimes itch occurs without these other findings, which can make the cause more difficult to identify and the treatment more complicated.

Itching of any cause may be acute (lasting less than six weeks) or chronic (lasting more than six weeks). If you experience acute itching when receiving certain anti-cancer medications, it may be a sign that you are having an allergic reaction, although this does not always mean that you cannot continue to receive the treatment. Cancer treatments associated with severe, chronic, or long-term itching include cetuximab, erlotinib, everolimus, gefitinib, interferon, interleukin-2, ipilimumab, panitumumab, radiation, stem cell transplants, and temsirolimus.

DID YOU KNOW?

All cancer treatments, including chemotherapy, targeted therapies, radiation, stem cell transplants, and even surgery (in the scar), can cause itching.

I was told that itching during treatment could indicate an allergy to my anti-cancer medicine. Does this mean I will have to stop my treatment?

Itching is just one of many signs and symptoms that indicate an allergy. An allergy occurs when the immune system is triggered by a medication, and can affect the skin and internal organs, including the lungs, liver, and kidneys. In addition to itch, an allergy may cause a rash, shortness of breath, fever, severe coughing, low blood pressure, sneezing, diarrhea, swelling (of the face, lips, or mouth), abdominal pain, or even losing consciousness. Many anti-cancer medications can cause itching, but that does not necessarily indicate you are allergic to the treatment. In fact, true allergies are rare with cancer medicines. If the itch is caused by a medicine, there are treatments against the itch that can be used so that the anti-cancer medicine can continue.

Itching Due to Cancer Medicines

All people who receive chemotherapy and targeted therapies react differently in terms of itching—some experience this side effect and others do not. If your skin feels itchy while you are receiving anti-cancer medications, it may be related to your medical history (such as allergies to other medicines or kidney and liver diseases), pre-existing dry skin, the chemotherapy or targeted therapy itself, or its dosage. Be sure to tell your doctor or nurse if you are experiencing any itching and whether you also have a rash or hives. In most cases, itch can be prevented or treated. Rarely do anti-cancer medicines need to be changed or stopped because of itch.

Where on the body the itching occurs will depend on the medication that is causing it. Twenty percent to 40 percent of those who receive cetuximab, cyclophosphamide, erlotinib, gefitinib, panitumumab, or sorafenib have an itchy scalp. Ipilimumab can cause itching on the legs or trunk. Itching from dasatinib and imatinib, interferon, lenalidomide, and tamoxifen, and most other medications occurs in the trunk. Docetaxel and paclitaxel may cause itch on the scalp and the back of the hands and feet. Itching from blood thinners occurs on the skin where they are injected (usually over the stomach or thighs). Capecitabine and doxorubicin can cause itching and burning on the palms and soles (otherwise known

Q My itching occurs mostly at night. What's the reason for this?

A Most people say that itching, of any cause, is more frequent at night when they are not as occupied with other activities. Therefore, try to stay engaged in some activity in the evenings so that your mind is not focused on your itch. Taking anti-itch medicines that cause drowsiness may also help when itching is worse at night. Medications such as diphenhydramine, doxepin, gabapentin, hydroxyzine, and pregabalin can help you sleep and decrease itch.

Medications That May Cause Itching

Antibiotics

Chemotherapies and targeted therapies

Actinomycin	Gefitinib	Pazopanib
Arsenic trioxide	Gemcitabine	Pemetrexed
Asparaginase	Ibritumomab	Procarbazine
ATRA	Imatinib	Retinoic acid
Bexarotene	Interferon alfa	Rituximab
Bleomycin	Interleukin-2	Romidepsin
Capecitabine	Ipilimumab	Sargramostim
Cetuximab	Irinotecan	Sorafenib
Chlorambucil	Lenalidomide	Streptozocin
Cladribine	Mechlorethamine	Temozolomide
Cyclophosphamide	Melphalan	Thalidomide
Cytarabine	Mercaptopurine	Thioguanine
Dasatinib	Methotrexate	Thiotepa
Daunorubicin	Nilotinib	Tositumomab
Docetaxel	Nilutamide	Vincristine
Doxorubicin	Octreotide	Vinorelbine
Erlotinib	Paclitaxel	Vorinostat
Etoposide	Panitumumab	

Hormone therapies

Anastrozole	Fluoxymesterone	Megestrol
Bicalutamide	Letrozole	Tamoxifen
Estramustine	Leuprolide	Toremifene
Exemestane	Medroxyprogesterone	

Blood thinners

Dalteparin	Tinzaparin
Enoxaparin	Warfarin

Blood stimulants

Darbepoetin alfa	Filgrastim	Pegfilgrastim
Epoetin alfa	Fondaparinux	

Morphine, codeine, or other opium derivatives

Nonsteroidal anti-inflammatory drugs

Aspirin	Ibuprofen	Naproxen

as hand-foot syndrome). Medicines to control cancer-related pain (codeine, morphine, and related ones) lead to itch in 30 percent of people. Those receiving chemotherapy or targeted therapies frequently develop dry skin, which can also itch. Itching with dryness is thought to be related to the medication's effects on sebaceous or sweat glands as well as on the normal growth of skin.

If itching is due to an allergic reaction, it develops within minutes to hours after receiving the medication and goes away quickly after it is stopped. On the other hand, itch that develops from dry skin often begins after several weeks of starting the culprit medication and can last for several weeks after stopping it. When itching is associated with dry skin, controlling the dryness will usually resolve the itch. When skin has a rash, or redness associated with itching, treating the rash or redness with topical steroids or oral anti-itch medicines and/or steroids will also improve the itching. If there is an allergy to a topically applied product such as an antibiotic cream or ointment, or to a dressing, removing it will help, but it is also important to treat with topical corticosteroid medications.

Itching Due to Radiation Therapy

Although you cannot feel radiation when it is given, it may cause a skin reaction two to three weeks after beginning treatment, with skin itching, burning, and pain. These symptoms may not improve for up to four to six weeks after the last treatment session. Itching related to radiation usually occurs at the site of the skin

Is there anything I can do to prevent the itch from radiation?

A recent study showed that by applying a topical corticosteroid cream (mometasone) daily from the first day of radiation, itching was reduced by about 30 percent. During radiation treatments, no creams or ointments should be applied to the area four hours before or after receiving radiation.

exposed to radiation and is more severe at the fifth or sixth week. The skin may become dry and red; there may be a burning sensation, followed by peeling. More than half of those receiving radiation report burning and itching. The good news is that there are effective ways of preventing and treating these symptoms.

Try not to scratch itchy skin because it could result in sores and infections. If your skin becomes irritated, it is important to treat the area with medicated creams or ointments (usually with corticosteroids or antibiotics) as soon as possible, since decreasing or stopping the radiation is usually not desirable in terms of making sure your radiation treatment is effective. Areas of the skin that involve friction and sweat, such as the underarms and under the breasts, may be more common sites of radiation-induced itching or irritation than other areas. Ideally, everyone receiving radiation for breast or head and neck cancers should apply a topical steroid cream (mometasone or betamethasone) daily, from the first day of treatment to the last.

DID YOU KNOW?
Scratching can lead to skin breakdown and infections, so it's best to avoid scratching and instead use anti-itch medications.

Itching and Surgery

Mild itching is a common and normal sign that a surgical wound is healing. This type of itch can last for several months, especially when the scar is forming. The reason

Q I've been applying a triple antibiotic and dressing my wound daily since my surgery two days ago. The area around the wound has become very rashy and itchy. Why is this happening?

A Fewer than five percent of surgical wounds become infected, and they are associated with pain, redness, swelling, and discharge after about the seventh day following surgery. Earlier reactions that occur within the first week, such as intense itch, are most likely an allergy to the sterilizing cleanser used by your surgeon, the tape used to secure the dressing, or a topical antibiotic. Triple antibiotics and those containing neomycin are a common cause of allergies.

Q I have been on chemotherapy for several months and have been doing very well. In the past week, I've started to itch everywhere. Am I allergic to the chemotherapy?

A Although anti-cancer medications are frequent causes of itch, there are a number of other possible causes: other drugs such as antibiotics, morphine, and codeine; dry skin; aging; the cancer itself; or liver, nerve, or kidney problems. Itching by itself does not represent an allergy, especially when it happens several months after starting chemotherapy or targeted therapies. Talk with your oncologist, but you should not stop taking your anti-cancer medicine unless he or she recommends it.

DID YOU KNOW?

Surgical wounds continue to heal for up to one year after surgery, and itching may be a normal part of this healing process.

healing wounds feel itchy is the growth of new cells underneath the scab or scar. As the cells continue to grow, they force the scab to expand, and the skin becomes tightly stretched. In particular, large problem scars (also known as keloids) can form several months after surgery and cause more itching. Body areas more susceptible to the formation of itchy, problem scars include the neck, upper chest and back, shoulders, and ears.

If you have surgery, your health care team will give you instructions on caring for wounds as they heal. To promote healing and prevent infections, avoid scratching the wound.

You should note that sometimes itching occurs as a result of the irritation from changing or removing bandages or can result from an allergy to the adhesives, bandages, or topical antibiotics. When taking bandages off, pull gently. Be sure to watch for signs of infection. It's normal to have some soreness, tenderness, tingling, numbness, and itching around the incision.

Scratching any part of the skin, including surgical wounds and scars, may increase the intensity of the itch and lead to infection. Because the skin's ability to protect the body is altered by both cancer and its treatments, skin infections are more common in people living with cancer. In addition, a weaker immune system can increase the risk of bacterial (staphylococcus), vi-

Q I've been taking over-the-counter diphenhydramine pills for itch, but they make me very sleepy. What can I do so I don't feel this way?

A Although effective, some anti-itch medicines lead to sedation, or sleepiness. One way to get around this problem is to take these medicines approximately one hour before going to sleep. This way, it will help you sleep and it will help relieve itch at night. Another possibility is to use an antihistamine during the day that does not make you sleepy, such as cetirizine, fexofenadine, or loratadine, which may be obtained over the counter.

ral (herpes and shingles), and fungal infections. With bacterial and fungal infections, itch usually occurs at the same time as the infection, along with swelling, redness, and pain. With viral infections, itch can occur before or during the appearance of the rash and can last for several months, even after the acute infection has gone away.

DID YOU KNOW?

Some ingredients in anti-itch creams and ointments, such as alcohol and lanolin, may cause irritation and allergies, so be sure to check with your doctor before buying them.

Ways to Treat the Itch

If you experience itching, it's best to tell members of your health care team so they can help you choose the treatment that is right for you. Before recommending a treatment, especially if the itch is over large areas of the body, your doctor or nurse may perform blood tests to check that your kidneys and liver are working normally and to find out whether the level of cells called eosinophils is high—an indication that an allergy is causing the itch. Because the chemicals histamine and serotonin are sometimes involved in itch, some treatments block the activity of these chemicals. When itch is caused directly by the underlying cancer, treating the cancer will relieve the itch.

Over-the-Counter Itch Fighters

Most people first turn to over-the-counter medications for itching—oral antihistamines such as diphen-hydramine or topical corticosteroids (such as hydrocortisone) or anti-itch creams containing benzocaine, lidocaine, menthol, or pramoxine. Although non-prescription medications may be an effective option, you should check with your health care team before using them. For example, medications such as over-the-counter hydrocortisone 1% (Cortizone-10, Cortaid) are the least potent steroids and are rarely permanently effective. Creams that have itch-fighting properties include Aveeno Calamine & Pramoxine HCl Anti-Itch Cream, Eucerin Skin Calming Itch-Relief Treatment, Lanacane Maximum Strength Anti-Itch Cream, Sarna Sensitive Anti-Itch Lotion, and Gold Bond Intensive Healing Anti-Itch Skin Protectant Cream. Oral antihistamines (diphenhydramine) may be useful in some cases of itching; some types do not cause drowsiness and can be used during the day (cetirizine, fexofenadine, loratadine).

Lukewarm and Colloidal Oatmeal Baths
Taking a bath in lukewarm water for no more than 15 minutes once a day or every other day may help relieve dry skin. Be aware that showering or bathing too often can aggravate dry skin, and hot water can promote itching. So be sure to test the water before you step into the tub or shower.

Using products such as Aveeno Skin Relief Bath Treatment and Skin Relief Shower and Bath Oil or RoBathol Bath Oil may help reduce itching and dryness. Many people find soaking in a tub reduces stress as well. Moisturizers added to the water at the end of a bath or applied to the skin after patting dry also help soothe itch. For information about the best moisturizers, see Chapter 3, "Taking Care of Dry Skin."

Soaps and Bathing Aids
Mild soaps contain reduced amounts of fragrances or detergents that can dry and irritate skin. Some good choices are soaps from Vanicream, Dove, Cetaphil, or Basis. Avoid using loofahs, sponges, or body scrubs because they can irritate the skin and are loaded with bacteria.

Topical Anti-itch Ingredients and Products

These ingredients and products should be used three to four times a day or as directed by your doctor:

Menthol An organic compound made synthetically or from peppermint or other mint oils, menthol gives a cooling sensation when applied to the skin and is available over the counter. Menthol has been used for many years and is usually present in many different creams in concentrations ranging from 1% to 3%. Some people living with cancer like menthol, others say they don't like the smell or that it makes them feel cold.

Diphenhydramine This medication is available over the counter as a cream that must be applied four times a day. However, it is not usually recommended as a topical medication because many people are allergic to it. Diphenhydramine is also available in pill form, which is effective and does not cause allergies, but it may cause drowsiness.

Doxepin This medicine is available in both topical and pill form. Both forms require prescriptions and are effective. Their main side effect is drowsiness, which can occur in 25 percent of people, even when used as a cream. For this reason, it should be applied in small amounts and for not more than one week at a time.

Pramoxine This topical anesthetic is usually combined with other anti-itch ingredients and provides relief for several hours. Other less frequently used anesthetics include benzocaine and lidocaine, which may cause allergies, so it's best to use them sparingly and for no more than several weeks at a time.

Salicylic acid This medication is most effective when itching is associated with thickened skin from rubbing or scratching. It is usually prescribed and mixed with other anti-itch medicines at a 1% to 3% concentration.

Corticosteroids When used properly, these medications can be a great tool to manage itch. The weakest type, hydrocortisone 1% cream, is sold over the counter. Anything stronger (and, therefore, more effective) requires a prescription and directions from your doctor.

Oral Anti-itch Medicines

Antihistamines These medicines are widely used and safe; they block histamine, a chemical involved in itch. Diphenhydramine and hydroxyzine are more potent but cause more drowsiness, so it's best to take them at night. During the day, non-sedating antihistamines to try include cetirizine, fexofenadine, and loratadine (all available over the counter). Common side effects include drowsiness, dry mouth and eyes, and urinary retention. Care must be taken when used by the elderly and those with glaucoma or a large prostate.

Doxepin This medication is both an antihistamine and an antidepressant. Its main side effect is drowsiness, and it should not be taken with other antidepressants. Dosage starts at 10 mg to 25 mg at bedtime and increased by 10 mg to 25 mg weekly as tolerated, for a maximum of 75 mg a day.

Gabapentin and pregabalin These medications are prescribed to treat pain, but their use has been expanded to treat itchy skin in difficult cases. They work by modulating the nerves. The dose of gabapentin is 300 mg to 1,800 mg a day in three divided doses. The pregabalin dose is 150 mg a day in two divided doses, which may be increased to a maximum of 450 mg a day. They must be used with caution in the elderly, and the dose has to be adjusted in people with kidney disease. The main side effects include drowsiness and leg swelling.

Corticosteroids These medications are effective anti-inflammatories. They decrease eosinophils, a type of blood cell that causes itchy skin. They work quickly and should not be taken for a long period. The most commonly used steroids are prednisone (at a dose of 20 mg to 40 mg a day) and dexamethasone (2 mg to 8 mg a day), depending on a person's weight. When given for longer than 10 days, they must be slowly decreased (or tapered) over several weeks.

Aprepitant is a medication originally developed to treat nausea and vomiting caused by chemotherapy. It also modulates certain nerves that are important for itching. It has been found that people suffering from severe itch related to their cancer or to a targeted therapy can improve remarkably with the use of aprepitant.

Itching: A Step-by-Step Guide to Treatment

Severity	Treatment
Grade 1 (mild, localized)	▪ Topical corticosteroids **AND** anti-itch creams three times daily ▪ Reassess in 2 weeks; if itch worsens or does not improve, proceed to next step
Grade 2 (moderate, intense, intermittent, affecting many parts of the body)	▪ Topical corticosteroids **AND** oral antihistamines three times daily ▪ Reassess in 2 weeks; if itch worsens or does not improve, proceed to next step
Grade 3 (severe, constant, affecting ability to sleep)	▪ Oral antihistamines **AND** oral corticosteroids (dexamethasone, prednisone), nerve modulators (aprepitant gabapentin, pregabalin) **OR** UV light therapy (phototherapy)

Prescription Therapies Against Itching: Taking the Next Step

If using over-the-counter medicines and changing bathing habits does not stop the itching, prescription medications (topical or oral) may be needed. In cases of infections causing itching, antibiotics, antifungals, or antivirals will help. These medications will be prescribed by your doctor depending on what part of your body has the infection and how severe it is. Your doctor may also recommend antihistamines (hydroxyzine), antidepressants (doxepin), or nerve modulators (aprepitant, gabapentin, pregabalin), since they block chemicals involved in itch. When you have widespread itch that resists treatment or experience itch with certain diseases such as mastocytosis, lymphomas, or leukemias, you may need to consult a dermatologist who can recommend ultraviolet (UV) light therapy (also called phototherapy). Shining this special light on your skin several times a week will help your dermatologist control your skin inflammation and itch. For itching on the scalp, your doctor can prescribe corticosteroids in

DID YOU KNOW?

The most common ingredients causing allergies are: nickel (a component of many metals), fragrances, neomycin (in antibiotic creams or ointments), balsam of Peru (in cosmetics and in certain foods and drinks), and thimerosal (a topical disinfectant).

shampoos (clobetasol, fluocinolone), liquids (clobetasol, fluocinonide), or foams (clobetasol, betamethasone).

A Final Reminder...

To prevent and treat itchy skin, you should moisturize daily, protect your skin from the sun, and use cleansing practices that do not dry out your skin. Remember that there are many ways to manage itch. When they are used together, your cancer treatment won't be interrupted, and you can live itch-free.

THINGS TO REMEMBER

- Tell your health care team if you are experiencing any itching and if you are using over-the-counter remedies to soothe the itch. It's important for your doctor or nurse to know whether the itch is associated with a rash or other skin changes (dryness, welts, etc.).

- Cancers that involve the skin (such as melanoma) or have spread to the skin (such as breast or ovarian cancer) commonly cause itching.

- Itching caused by an allergy usually occurs within minutes to hours after a chemotherapy infusion or ingestion.

- Itching caused by radiation treatment may occur five to six weeks after treatment begins and may take four to six weeks to go away once treatment is complete. It can be prevented with the use of a topical corticosteroid.

- Itching is a common sign that a surgical wound is healing. To promote healing and prevent infection, avoid scratching the wound area.

- Even if your anti-cancer therapy is causing itching, it can usually be managed so that you can continue receiving treatment.

- There are many ways to treat itch, from over-the-counter to prescription medications, used topically or orally.

CHAPTER 5

Keeping Nails Healthy

When most people begin chemotherapy, they're not likely to think about their nails. In fact, many people are surprised to learn that chemotherapy can affect the fingernails and toenails. Although nail problems are not a common side effect of most anti-cancer drugs, they can occur more often with certain types of medicines, especially the so-called targeted treatments and taxane chemotherapies (paclitaxel and docetaxel).

These changes can occur in all or in just some of the nails. Some of these side effects are simply annoying, whereas others can be more severe and require treatment. They may involve only the nails, cuticles, or nail folds as well. Nail changes caused by anti-cancer drugs are usually temporary and may improve even as treatment continues or after it is finished. However, because nails grow slowly, it may take months for them to return to normal. So it is ideal to prevent problems before they happen or as soon as they arise.

DID YOU KNOW?

Nails are solid structures made from a skin protein known as keratin, and dried, flattened skin cells (similar to claws in animals).

My nails started changing color and texture with the cancer treatment. Will they go back to normal?

Yes. Nail changes from cancer treatments are usually temporary, although it may take several months after treatment before they go back to normal. Fingernails grow nearly four times faster than toenails, and men's nails grow faster than women's.

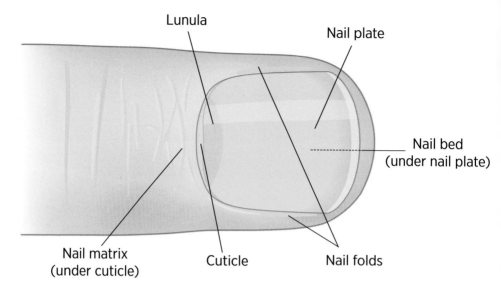

ANATOMY OF A NAIL
The nail is composed of several parts: the nail plate (the hard surface), lunula (half moon-shaped white part), nail bed (skin under the nail), cuticle, matrix (which forms the plate), and the nail folds (skin overlapping the nail).

Before starting chemotherapy, be sure to ask your health care team whether nail changes are likely to occur from the medications you will receive. This will ensure that you can maintain the health of your nails so that they look and feel as good as possible during treatment.

How Nails Are Affected by Treatments

There are several types of nail changes that can result from anti-cancer treatments. Most of them are mild and only affect the appearance of the nail, whereas others can be more severe and can cause discomfort or pain. The types of nail changes depend on the medicine that is given and the duration of treatment. By far, brittleness is the most common side effect and can be caused by any chemotherapy or after stem cell transplants.

Depending on what specific part of the nail is affected, different types of changes can occur. If the nail matrix (see illustration above) is affected, nails will be brittle and have grooves, ridges, or white or dark discoloration.

Nail bed problems result in pain under the nail; red, purple, or green discoloration, with separation or lifting of the nail; and possibly even infections. When nail folds or cuticles are affected, there is pain, redness, and swelling—ingrown nails and even infections may also occur.

Other nail changes include bleeding underneath the fingernails or toenails, known as subungual hemorrhage, and skin infections around or under the nails, called paronychia. Sometimes, nail infections are first noticed when the skin around the nails becomes red and swells because of excess fluid. These infections can cause the affected nails to become sore and tender, making it difficult to perform daily activities. In some cases, pus leaks from the infected nails. Be sure to inform your health care team at the first sign of red, tender nails, as they may indicate an infection that needs to be treated with oral antibiotics (such as cephalexin or ciprofloxacin).

In most people, nail changes caused by anti-cancer therapies begin within two to three months of starting treatments and improve within a few months afterward. People generally do not lose their nails but may have thickening or discoloration for several months after finishing treatment. In these cases, it is important to rule out a persistent fungal nail infection, which may occur after nails are injured or damaged by chemotherapy.

If you experience nail changes, it's important to remember that they are a temporary, reversible reaction to your cancer treatment. Generally, the nail goes back to normal.

DID YOU KNOW?

Nails play an important role in supporting, protecting, and adding sensation to tissues in fingers and toes and in helping to hold and handle objects.

How Anti-Cancer Treatments Affect Nails

Part of Nail Affected	Result
Matrix	Grooves, white lines, and brittle nails
Bed	Brown or white discoloration, lifting, or loss, and infections
Folds or cuticles	Inflammation, infections, separation, and pain

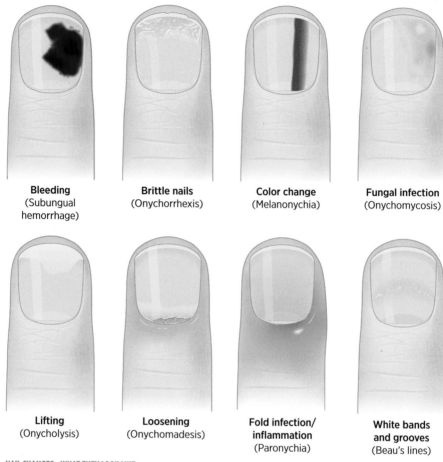

Bleeding (Subungual hemorrhage)	**Brittle nails** (Onychorrhexis)	**Color change** (Melanonychia)	**Fungal infection** (Onychomycosis)
Lifting (Onycholysis)	**Loosening** (Onychomadesis)	**Fold infection/ inflammation** (Paronychia)	**White bands and grooves** (Beau's lines)

NAIL CHANGES : WHAT THEY LOOK LIKE
The various nail changes can sometimes develop at the same time in one nail or in several nails at a time. The medical term for each change is included in parenthesis.

Which Anti-Cancer Medications May Cause Most Nail Problems?

Although any chemotherapy can affect the nails, some of the so-called targeted therapies (cetuximab, erlotinib, lapatinib, panitumumab), as well as some conventional chemotherapies (docetaxel, paclitaxel), tend to cause more side effects in the nails. One study on the chemotherapy docetaxel found that nail changes occurred in about 80 percent of people, with up to 30 percent having tenderness or infections that limited their daily activities. Docetaxel and paclitaxel, in par-

Anti-Cancer Treatments Associated With Nail Changes

Nail Change	May Be Caused By
Separation of the nail from the nail bed	Capecitabine, docetaxel, doxorubicin, eribulin, etoposide, ixabepilone, mercaptopurine, methotrexate, mitoxantrone, paclitaxel
Bleeding underneath the nails	Docetaxel, paclitaxel, sorafenib, sunitinib
Discolored nails (white or dark lines)	Bleomycin, cyclophosphamide, dacarbazine, daunorubicin, docetaxel, doxorubicin, erlotinib, etoposide, fluorouracil, gefitinib, idarubicin, imatinib, lapatinib, melphalan, paclitaxel, panitumumab, topotecan, vincristine
Skin infection under/around the nails	Cetuximab, docetaxel, eribulin, erlotinib, gefitinib, lapatinib, paclitaxel, panitumumab
Redness/swelling of skin around the nails	Cetuximab, eribulin, erlotinib, gefitinib, lapatinib, panitumumab
Grooves/ridges/brittle nails	Any chemotherapy, graft-versus-host disease
Nail loss	Docetaxel, paclitaxel, graft-versus-host disease

ticular, appear to cause nail changes more often than other types of chemotherapy. People who receive these medications may notice darkening underneath their nails and/or separation of the nail from the skin.

Although there is no proven way to prevent nail changes from these chemotherapies, there are ways that can help reduce the damage. According to clinical studies, people whose fingernails and toenails were kept cold before and after chemotherapy sessions with docetaxel had fewer and less severe problems with their nails and the nearby skin than those who did not use the cold technique.

Called cold glove/sock therapy, this approach uses a special frozen glove or slipper. The theory is that less of the blood (and the chemotherapy) reach-

DID YOU KNOW?

Taking 2.5 mg (or 2,500 mcg) of vitamin B$_7$ (biotin) can make nails stronger and grow faster.

es these colder areas, so fewer side effects should result. The gloves are worn before, during, and after chemotherapy (for a total of approximately one-and-a-half hours). Halfway through the session, a new frozen glove is used to ensure that the nails remain cold. One study found that among people who wore the gloves, nearly 90 percent had no nail problems. Researchers call these results "striking" and will continue to study this frozen glove treatment (and frozen socks for the feet).

Although most nail side effects from chemotherapy are not severe, sometimes they can lead to painful infections that emit a bad odor. That is why it is so important to tell your health care team about any nail changes. Your doctor or nurse can help treat nail effects and make sure that your cancer treatment can continue.

After two to three months of treatment with the "targeted" chemotherapies, about 50 percent of people experience inflamed and reddened skin around the fingernails and toenails. This condition is easily confused with ingrown toenails. If it is left untreated, the pain may continue, and the nail as well as the folds may become infected.

Other anti-cancer medicines that may cause nail changes include sorafenib and sunitinib (both taken orally). People who receive these medicines can experience bleeding underneath the nails, which looks like tiny dark brown lines or dirt (but it is not actual dirt). This side effect may occur as a result of how this type of drug works to fight cancer—by affecting blood vessels. Usually, no particular treatment is needed, but a dark nail polish may be used to hide the discoloration.

Making Brittle Nails Better

During and after treatment, caring for your nails is very important. By following the tips below, you can make nail care a part of your regular health plan.

Take your vitamins and supplements. Strong, healthy nails depend on vitamin B_7 (biotin). Be sure to take at least 2.5 mg (2,500 mcg) every day along with orthosilicic acid, 10 mg a day (BioSil, 1 capsule twice daily). Keep in mind that you can start taking these supplements right after you finish your course of treatment. Most oncologists do not allow the use of these supplements while you are still in treatment with chemotherapy or radiation therapy, since it is not known whether they can interfere with their efficacy. Be sure to talk with your doctor before taking any over-the-counter supplements or medications.

Take care when cutting your nails. Trimming nails straight across helps avoid ingrown toenails. If you are experiencing nail problems, or it is difficult to cut your nails, it may be time to visit a podiatrist. You can find one at the American Podiatric Medical Association (www.apma.org).

Dry hands and feet thoroughly. After washing dishes, swimming, or taking a bath or shower, dry your fingers and toes well to avoid fungal infections. You may consider wearing plastic or vinyl gloves when

DID YOU KNOW?

Due to the slow growth of nails, it may take several weeks for nail changes to first appear. It takes about six months to regrow a complete fingernail and about 12 to 18 months to regrow a toenail.

Preventive Care for Nails

Keep nails trimmed and clean, but avoid salon manicures or pedicures during your treatment.

Wear vinyl gloves when cleaning the house, washing dishes, or gardening. For even more protection, buy vinyl gloves one size larger and wear white cotton gloves underneath, to absorb sweat and cushion the nails and fingertips.

Pay special attention to your cuticles:
- Do not bite away dry cuticles or hangnails.
- Do use cuticle remover cream or gel to prevent nail dryness and splitting.

Do not bite your nails or use them as tools. File them gently.

Take 2.5 mg (2,500 mcg) of vitamin B_7 (biotin) and 10 mg of orthosilicic acid (BioSil) every day to make nails grow stronger and faster.

Tell your doctor or nurse about any signs of skin infection around the nails.

Adapted from www.breastcancer.org/treatment/side_effects/nail_changes.jsp

Q I have been on lapatinib for breast cancer for the past year. My nails have become ingrown and painful, and my doctor applied silver nitrate and asked me to apply a povidone-iodine ointment daily. It is helping, but it left this dark discoloration. Is there anything I can do for this?

A Silver nitrate application is a simple and effective way to treat infections caused by cetuximab, erlotinib, lapatinib, and panitumumab. Usually, the tip of the applicator is soaked in tap water and then applied to the inflamed nail folds. Your doctor may also recommend daily application of a povidone-iodine ointment. Dark or yellow discoloration will remain and can be concealed by using dark nail polish, such as OPI Lincoln Park After Dark or Black Cherry Chutney, China Glaze Evening Seduction, Sally Hansen Pat on the Black, or Polished Mama Date Night.

DID YOU KNOW?

Although most anti-cancer medications can affect your nails, so can poor eating or nutrition. As a result of poor nutrition, the nails grow more slowly and become brittle.

washing dishes or doing housework. Wearing white cotton gloves underneath ensures that moisture and sweat won't irritate your skin and nails.

Don't drown your nails. It sounds strange, but constantly submerging your nails in water can actually dry them out.

Wear all-cotton socks. Cotton socks help absorb dampness and may help avoid fungal nail infections and athlete's foot.

Buff your nails. This can increase the blood supply to the nails, which helps them grow and stay strong.

Keep cuticles healthy. Rubbing a little bit of petroleum jelly (Vaseline) or cream into your cuticles and the skin around your nails can help keep them moisturized.

Use a clear coat of polish or nail strengthener/hardener. Not only does a coat of nail polish prolong the life of a manicure, it also protects the nails and strengthens brittle nails. NailTek has natural products that fill ridges (NailTek Foundation) and strengthen nails (NailTek II: Intensive Therapy for soft peeling nails and NailTek III: Protection Plus for dry, brittle nails).

Remember, nail hardeners with up to 2% formalin, which is not the same as formaldehyde, may also provide an additional benefit. Apply two top coats after applying nail polish, and apply one coat of nail strengthener daily (CITRA Formaldehyde-Free #3; OPI Nail Envy Natural Nail Strengthener; China Glaze Nail Strengthener & Growth Formula; Sally Hansen Hard As Nails Strengthener). You may apply a top coat of strengthener daily, even over nails with polish.

For tears in the tips of the nails, use IBD 5-Second Professional Nail Glue. Apply one drop on the torn nail, and hold pressure for five seconds, then allow to set for one minute.

Avoid toxic nail products. Be sure to select nail products that do not contain these harmful chemicals: toluene, formaldehyde, or dibutyl phthalate; OPI, China Glaze, Sally Hansen, Zoya, and Polished Mama are good products to use as nail polish.

If the nails are peeling, trim the tip, then buff the surface of the tip with a file, in one direction, away from the nail matrix.

Do not use acrylic nails. Acrylics tend to weaken your natural nails and make them brittle. Instead, use

Q Can I get a manicure or pedicure at my nail salon during treatment? If not, how soon after treatment can I start getting one again?

A Salons pose a risk for anyone: an infection can be picked up from other people's utensils and basins. Since most chemotherapies temporarily weaken the immune system, your chance of getting these infections may be higher. However, you can carefully cut your nails and cuticles at home, with the help of a friend or family member, and use nail polish. Once you finish treatment and your immune system is back to normal, you can return to the nail salon. How long it takes for the immune system to bounce back fully depends on the chemotherapy used and your overall health, but it ranges from two to three months.

I want to avoid as many chemicals as possible. What nail polish should I use?

Dark nail polishes are good because they hide any nail color changes from chemotherapy. In general, a water-based nail polish is ideal, since it contains the least amount of chemicals. Use brands that are free of dibutyl phthalate, toluene, and formaldehyde, the so-called three-free polishes. They include OPI, China Glaze, Sally Hansen, Zoya, and Polished Mama.

DID YOU KNOW?

Dark lines or spots in the nail can be caused by chemotherapy and can stay for up to 6 months after treatment. There is no way of removing them, so use a nail polish dark enough to hide them.

silk wraps applied at a salon, which can give the appearance of stronger nails. If you have acrylics now, remove them and give your nails a few months' rest to help them regain their strength. For exposed skin of the nail bed from a torn nail, cover with Micropore medical tape in the shape of the missing part of the nail.

Pay attention to your cuticles. Cuticles protect the roots of your nails from harmful bacteria, so never cut them; just gently push them back when they are moist. Avon Nail Experts Instant Gel Cuticle Remover melts away the cuticles quickly with no cutting or pushing. A natural cuticle softener alternative is olive oil: apply a few drops, leave on for 5–10 minutes, then wipe off.

When the nail folds are red or inflamed, use specially made bandages that have a smooth gel covering. A good product is Gel Tube Toe/Finger Bandages and Toe-Aid Dressings from Southwest Medical.

When brittle nails are painful, your doctor may also prescribe the vitamin A cream tazarotene. When it is applied twice daily to nails and folds, these brittle nails get tougher.

For cracked nails, use Calico Invisible Nail Bandages or Crack Attacker Instant Repair Nail Bandages or have silk wraps applied at a salon.

Use natural nail polish removers, such as Honeybee Gardens Odorless Nail Polish Remover, Suncoat Natural Nail Polish Remover, Dr.'s REMEDY Non-Acetone Enriched Nail Polish Remover.

Nailing Nail Changes

Although most nail changes caused by anti-cancer medicines are temporary, your doctor may need to deal with the more troublesome nail changes to help you cope with the rest of your cancer treatment. Fortunately, there are several effective ways to manage these nail conditions.

Nail infections usually do not go away unless they are treated. That's why it's important to tell your doctor or nurse if you have signs of a nail infection, so the appropriate antibiotic can be given. It is always a good idea for the doctor to swab the area or clip a tiny piece of the nail to prescribe the correct antibiotic or antifungal medicine. At home, it's a good idea to soak infected fingers or toes in a solution of equal parts white vinegar and lukewarm or cool water for 15 minutes twice daily until the symptoms improve. An alternative is to add one teaspoon of bleach in a foot basin or similar container. These antiseptic solutions will destroy bacteria and dry any oozing areas.

Nail Changes After Stem Cell Transplants

Many people with cancers of the blood or lymph nodes are treated with stem cell transplants. These lifesaving treatments replace cancerous blood cells with newer, healthy blood cells from a donor. Sometimes, transplanted cells from a donor see the recipient's body as "foreign" and attack the skin, intestines, or liver. This may be a serious complication that doctors call graft-versus-host disease (GVHD). GVHD can occur shortly after transplantation or even years later.

GVHD can cause changes in the nails. Symptoms include long, colored streaks across the nails and roughness, ridging, splitting, and even loss of the nails if left untreated. Since these changes are a result of treatable forms of GVHD, it is important to address them promptly.

If you have had or are planning to have a transplant, be sure to pay special attention to your nails. Let your health care team know about any changes in your nails, as they may be a sign of GVHD. (See Chapter 9, "Stem Cell Transplants and Your Skin," for more detailed information on how transplants can affect your skin.)

Q I finished my chemotherapy one year ago, but my nails are still brittle. Is there any nail polish that can make them look better?

A Yes—nail polish gels, which come in many different colors, last longer (two to three weeks) and make nails less likely to chip or break. They are applied in salons, and just like an ordinary manicure, the cuticles are pushed and nails filed and buffed. But then, two or three layers of gel polish are applied. In between each one, the polish is "dried" under a special UV light. Shellac and Dashing Diva Gelife are two of the most popular brands found at salons. They may be more expensive than a regular manicure/pedicure but last much longer, and your nails will look perfect. Remember to cover the skin on your hands with a cloth, sunscreen, or glove when using UV lights to dry the nail polish.

DID YOU KNOW?

The pink color of nails comes from blood vessels in the skin underneath—the nails are translucent (semi-transparent).

Treating Infections

Once changes in your nail occur, the risk of infection may increase, especially if the nails become loose or there is any redness or swelling in the skin around the nails. Infections under and around the nails are more frequently caused by cetuximab, docetaxel, erlotinib, lapatinib, paclitaxel, and panitumumab. So be sure to alert your health care team if, during treatment, you notice any signs of a nail infection.

Using a topical antibiotic (Polysporin or mupirocin) or an antiseptic (povidone-iodine) ointment daily is a good way to fight off nail infections early on. If the infection is painful, your doctor may prescribe a two-week course of oral antibiotics such as cephalexin or ciprofloxacin.

Nail Infections: Signs and Symptoms

Pain at rest or when holding objects

Green or yellow discoloration under the nails

Oozing of foul-smelling fluid from under the nails

Redness, swelling, or "pus pockets" around the nail

Nail Infections (Paronychia): A Step-by-Step Guide to Treatment

Severity	Treatment
Grade 1 (mild)	▪ Chemotherapy can be continued at the same dose/frequency ▪ Daily application of topical antibiotic (Polysporin, mupirocin) **OR** antiseptic (povidone-iodine) ointment ▪ Reassess in 2 weeks; if it worsens or does not improve, proceed to the next step
Grade 2 (moderate)	▪ Chemotherapy can be continued at the same dose/frequency ▪ Oral antibiotics (cephalexin, ciprofloxacin) **AND** topical antiseptic (povidone-iodine) ointment **AND** chemical cauterization or cryotherapy by a dermatologist ▪ Reassess in 2 weeks; if it worsens or does not improve, proceed to the next step
Grade 3 (severe)	▪ Chemotherapy may be interrupted or decreased by your oncologist ▪ Oral antibiotics (cephalexin, ciprofloxacin) **AND** partial/complete nail removal or chemical cauterization or cryotherapy by a dermatologist ▪ Reassess in 2 weeks; if it worsens or does not improve, your oncologist may change or decrease chemotherapy

If a fungal infection is diagnosed, treatment includes a topical (ciclopirox and econazole) or oral antifungal (terbinafine, itraconazole). Fungal nail infections improve slowly, so antifungal treatment needs to continue for at least 3 months. Some treatments require blood tests to make sure your liver is not affected by the medications. People with cancer or other diseases of the liver usually cannot receive systemic antifungal treatments.

If the nail folds become inflamed, your doctor may use the chemical silver nitrate, which comes in the

Q How do I know if my nails are infected?

A Signs of infection include redness, swelling, and pain around the nails, sometimes with a discharge of foul-smelling fluid. About 30 to 50 percent of patients who receive treatments such as cetuximab, docetaxel, erlotinib, lapatinib, paclitaxel, or panitumumab develop a skin infection around the nails, called paronychia. This infection usually begins two to three months after the start of treatment but can occur as late as six months afterward. Any fingernail or toenail can be affected, and the infection needs to be treated, even if chemotherapy has finished.

DID YOU KNOW?

Daily application of the antiseptic ointment povidone-iodine is a good way to stop nail infections as soon as they begin. It is available over the counter in pharmacies or online.

tip of a long matchstick-like applicator. When applied to affected areas, silver nitrate cauterizes, or burns, the infection and the inflamed tissues. Alternatives to chemical cauterization include cryotherapy, in which a dermatologist sprays the area with a very cold liquid that destroys damaged tissues around the nail. This is particularly useful for nail fold infections called paronychia, which are caused by the targeted treatments cetuximab, erlotinib, lapatinib, and panitumumab.

Silver nitrate chemical cauterization can improve paronychia and is used before considering removal of the entire nail surgically (called nail avulsion). Removing parts of the nail is a procedure done by a dermatologist when the infection becomes painful, limiting the ability to perform daily activities or walk. Using silver nitrate can cause parts of the nails and surrounding skin to turn a dark color. There may also be some minor stinging, which lasts a few minutes after the application.

THINGS TO REMEMBER

- Nail changes caused by chemotherapy are usually temporary; they improve once treatment is completed. The only changes that may persist are infections, which must be treated with antibiotics or antifungals.

- Most nail side effects are cosmetic, involving changes in the color and texture of fingernails and toenails. Rarely are they more severe, involving separation or lifting of the nails or infections.

- Certain anti-cancer medications are more likely to cause nail changes than others, especially taxanes (docetaxel and paclitaxel) and "targeted" treatments (cetuximab, erlotinib, gefitinib, and panitumumab).

- Nail infections may require oral or topical antibiotics or antifungals, or procedures by a dermatologist, such as chemical cauterization, cryotherapy, or nail avulsion.

- Special frozen gloves and slippers worn during chemotherapy with docetaxel seem to be an effective way to reduce side effects on nails.

- Be sure to inform your health care team at the first sign of red, tender nails, which may indicate an infection.

- Soaking infected nails in a solution of white vinegar (diluted in equal amounts with water) or bleach (one teaspoon in 2 gallons of water) will help destroy bacteria and dry out areas discharging fluid.

- Using nail strengtheners and vitamin supplements can keep nails strong and healthy long after treatment is over.

- Stem cell transplants can also affect the nails. If untreated, these nail problems could be permanent, so be sure to inform your doctor of any changes.

CHAPTER 6

Handling Hair Changes

One of the most well-known side effects of anti-cancer treatments is hair loss, what doctors call alopecia. For many women and men, hair loss can be one of the most distressing side effects they experience. If you are concerned about potential or current hair loss, you are not alone—in surveys of women with breast cancer, hair loss is ranked as one of the top five most important side effects, behind nausea and vomiting. Some women feel that losing their hair is worse than losing a breast. In fact, eight percent of women say they would reject chemotherapy solely on the basis of possible hair loss.

Studies show that people older than age 60 appear to be more affected than those who are younger, perhaps an unexpected finding. How people are affected by hair loss may depend on their type of cancer. For instance, it is the second most important side effect for people with breast or lung cancer, but those with gastrointestinal cancers do not even name it as one of their top 10 concerns. In people with cancers that are more advanced, hair loss may be less important, according to another study.

Many people find hair loss to be psychologically and emotionally trying, causing frustration and anxiety. One difference between men and women is that men tend to be more concerned about hair loss on their body than on their scalp.

DID YOU KNOW?

The fastest growing tissue in the body is hair. There are approximately 100,000 hairs in the scalp and 5 million hairs on the body.

Q **After chemotherapy, will I regrow all of my hair, and will it look and feel the same as it did before treatment?**

A Although most people regrow a full head of hair after losing it during chemotherapy, it's impossible to predict what will happen for each individual after treatment. Persistent hair thinning rarely happens in people whose treatment included busulfan or taxanes (paclitaxel or docetaxel), prior radiation therapy, or a stem cell transplant that resulted in graft-versus-host disease. If your hair does not grow back, your doctor can check for other conditions that can lead to hair loss such as vitamin D, thyroid hormone, or iron deficiency, for example.

DID YOU KNOW?

Hair on the scalp grows about half an inch (or 1.3 centimeters) every month. Each hair lasts between two and six years.

Until they are faced with its possible loss, many people do not realize just how much their hair is tied to their self-image. Some people are concerned with a loss of privacy, since a bald head may signal to others that they are receiving chemotherapy for cancer.

Whatever you may feel about hair loss, it's important to remember that it is usually temporary, and the hair *will* grow back. When asked one year after treatment, the quality of life for women with breast cancer was the same for those who received chemotherapy and had hair loss as for those who did not. People deal with hair loss in one of two ways: by not paying attention to it or by hiding their baldness under a wig, scarf, turban, or hat. Either way, if people are prepared for it, they usually adjust to the hair loss and are able to receive chemotherapy with self-confidence and strength. Support from family and friends can go a long way toward making the best of a difficult situation. And when the situation can't be avoided, adjusting your thinking about the situation can help: it's a new look that will change over time.

This chapter will help you learn what to expect in terms of possible hair loss and changes and some simple steps to help you cope. Being prepared in this way reduces the negative impact of hair loss and helps build a sense of control.

Anti-Cancer Medications and Hair Loss (or Thinning)

Rapidly growing cancer cells are the main targets of chemotherapy. Although these medicines are destroying cancer cells, they often affect other healthy, fast-growing cells in the body, including those that make hair grow. When the structures that form the hair (the hair follicles) are affected by chemotherapy, radiation, or other medications, the hair stops growing or grows more slowly. Many of these powerful anti-cancer treatments can cause hair to thin, fall out in patches, or fall out completely. Hair loss or slowing of hair growth can occur anywhere on the body, including the head, face, arms, legs, underarms, and pubic area. It sometimes starts with a tingling, perhaps tender feeling, as the first strands come out. The loss of hair may be sudden or gradual but with each chemotherapy cycle (and especially after the second one), the rate of hair loss increases. You may notice loose hair on your pillow, in your hairbrush, or in the drains of the sink or shower. Generally, hair loss from chemotherapy is not permanent, but hair can grow back with a different texture (the so-called chemo curls) and in some cases with a different color.

The potential loss of your hair—and the potential amount—during chemotherapy depend on several factors. The type of chemotherapy and how it is given (in terms of dose and frequency) can affect the amount of hair a person may lose. Different doses of chemotherapy can cause varying degrees of hair loss, from just thinning to complete baldness.

> **DID YOU KNOW?**
> Some studies have shown that hair loss affects men as much, or sometimes even more, than women.

Q **My hair has been thinning as a result of a treatment I am on. Will washing my hair make it fall out faster?**

A There are about 100,000 hairs on the scalp, and people normally lose about 100 hairs every day. Hair becomes fragile during chemotherapy and may fall out more easily during washing or combing.

Some chemotherapies have been linked more strongly to hair loss than others (see box on next page). Moreover, hormonal therapies, used to treat some breast, endometrial, neuroendocrine, and prostate cancers, may also cause hair thinning. These medications are intended to stop or alter the effect of hormones that help some tumors grow, such as estrogen or testosterone. Anti-estrogen drugs such as tamoxifen and the aromatase inhibitors anastrozole, exemestane, and letrozole can thin the hair on the scalp, increase hairs on the face, and even darken hair color. If you notice thinning hair from hormonal therapy, it should start to thicken again within a few weeks after treatment is over. However, people with certain types of cancer often must take hormonal treatments for years. After the end of treatment, it may take a few months before you really notice the difference in your hair.

Aside from hair loss, about 60 percent of people treated with standard chemotherapies such as cytarabine, dactinomycin, doxorubicin, and etoposide will have some type of change to the texture of their hair. For instance, curly hair may grow back straight, and dark hair may grow in lighter or gray (and vice versa). This change is often temporary, but can be permanent in some.

It is important to remember that not all chemotherapies cause hair loss. Standard chemotherapies

I'll be starting treatment next week, and my oncologist said that it's the type of chemotherapy that causes significant hair loss. When will my hair start falling out, and do you recommend I shave it or just let it fall on its own?

After the first two cycles, your hair will start falling out. Because hairs on the scalp are in different stages of growth, they will fall out in clumps. So most people recommend shaving the hair all at once after the first cycle. This may be less traumatic than seeing bald spots develop or the hair falling off in pieces. Your oncologist can talk with you about whether there are other effective chemotherapy options that might not affect the hair as much.

Anti-Cancer Medicines That May Cause Hair Loss

Mild

Arsenic trioxide	Fludarabine	Procarbazine
Bexarotene	Fluorouracil	Streptozocin
Bleomycin	Gemcitabine	Sunitinib
Carmustine (BCNU)	Hydroxyurea	Temozolomide
Capecitabine	Interferon	Thalidomide
Chlorambucil	Interleukin	Thioguanine
Cisplatin	L-Asparaginase	Thiotepa
Cyclophosphamide	Mercaptopurine	Trastuzumab
Dacarbazine	Melphalan	Vemurafenib
Dasatinib	Methotrexate	
Estramustine	Nilotinib	

Moderate

Actinomycin	Irinotecan	Topotecan
ATRA	Mechlorethamine	Vinblastine
Busulfan	Mitomycin	Vincristine
Cetuximab	Mitoxantrone	Vinorelbine
Dactinomycin	Panitumumab	Vorinostat
Erlotinib	Sorafenib	
Floxuridine	Teniposide	

Severe

Cytarabine	Doxorubicin	Ifosfamide
Daunorubicin	Etoposide	Paclitaxel
Docetaxel	Idarubicin	Vindesine

that do not usually cause hair loss include carboplatin, carmustine, cisplatin, and fludarabine. Some of the newer, targeted therapies are less likely to cause hair loss than many of the traditional chemotherapies. The targeted therapies include cetuximab, dasatinib, erlotinib, imatinib, lapatinib, nilotinib, panitumumab, sorafenib, sunitinib, vandetanib, and vemurafenib. With these newer types of treatment, some hair thinning and hair loss may occur, but it almost always is reversible, even when people continue to receive the medicine.

Hair Care Suggestions

Before Treatment

Cut it short. A shorter hairstyle now may help make hair loss less noticeable later, and you might like the change.

Consider a "cover-up." Wigs, scarves, turbans, and hats come in many styles, so now might be a good time to find one you like, unless you decide not to wear anything at all on your head.

During Treatment

Shave it off. If your scalp becomes sensitive as hair begins to fall out, consider shaving your head. If you choose to wear a wig, a shaved head makes it more comfortable to do so.

Protect what remains. Using a satin pillowcase, a soft hairbrush, or gentle shampoo may help your sensitive scalp.

After Treatment

Be patient and optimistic. Hair often grows back slowly, or at least more slowly than you would like. It also may have a different color or texture than before, but just like you, hair takes time to heal from cancer treatments.

Be gentle with your new hair. New hair can be fragile and may be damaged by styling and blow drying, especially with hot air. Give it time to grow and become strong before having it colored or permed.

Adapted from www.mayoclinic.com/health/hair-loss

DID YOU KNOW?

More than half of your hair has to be lost before other people can notice it.

Rarely, people living with cancer will have hair loss that is not due to the anti-cancer treatment, but rather to the cancer directly involving the skin on the scalp, a condition called alopecia neoplastica. This condition has been seen in people with breast, cervical, colon, stomach, and endometrial cancers, as well as skin lymphomas. Women with breast cancer represent 80 percent of people who have this type of hair loss, and if it does occur, it happens about 5 years after the initial diagnosis. Alopecia neoplastica presents with bald, red patches or bumps that do not itch or hurt. Treatment consists of anti-cancer medications (ideally a type that

How soon after I finish chemotherapy can I start dyeing my hair? And if I am getting chemotherapy that doesn't cause hair loss, can I use hair dye?

 Doctors generally recommend waiting until your hair is about an inch long before coloring it. Because hair doesn't start growing until two or three months after chemotherapy, it could take about two to four months for your hair to reach that length. If the type of anti-cancer therapy you are getting does not result in hair loss, there is no reason why you can't use hair dyes. Inform your doctor if your scalp becomes sensitive or irritated at any point. You may want to use chemical-free or vegetable-based dyes at first. Do not, however, dye your eyelashes or eyebrows.

does not cause additional hair loss) and possibly surgical removal of the bald areas.

Dealing With Excess Facial Hair

Surprisingly, up to two thirds of people on certain medications (cetuximab, corticosteroids, erlotinib, gefitinib, panitumumab) experience more hair growth on the face (including eyelashes, eyebrows, and beard area). You can use an electric razor (such as the Panasonic Pivoting Head Facial Trimmer), threading at a salon, electrolysis (find a licensed electrologist from the International Guild of Professional Electrologists at [800] 830-3247 or at www.igpe.org), or laser treatments (done by a dermatologist or plastic surgeon). Avoid chemical hair removers (such as Nair or Neet) and waxing, as they may cause irritation and burning. For bushy and out-of-control eyebrows, you can also use an eyebrow trimmer (Noxzema or Personna Eyebrow Trimmer and Shaper). These tiny disposable razors are ideal for shaving and shaping bushy eyebrows, easy to use, and inexpensive.

The cream eflornithine has been approved for the treatment of unwanted facial hair, and when applied twice daily is able to slow hair growth. Changes are noticeable within two to six months, and most people

DID YOU KNOW?

Some types of chemotherapy can make your hair lighter or darker. These changes are usually reversible, and your hair will go back to its normal color several months after treatment. If you don't like the color changes, it is safe for you to dye it.

The Cost of Unwanted Hair

Choose the hair removal option that's best for you, based on these factors:

Method	Location	Cost	Time Needed/ Frequency	Irritation	Potentially Permanent	Comments
Shaving	Home	Low	Short/frequent	Low	No	Consider electric razors
Plucking	Home	Low	Long/frequent	Moderate	No	Uncomfortable and time-consuming
Threading	Salon	Low	Short/ infrequent	Low- moderate	No	Highly recommended; find a threading salon in your area
Eflornithine cream	Home	High	Short/frequent	Low	No	Still need to remove hair since cream will only slow hair growth
Laser	Doctor's office	High	Long/ infrequent	Moderate	Yes	Need to repeat several times; specific lasers for people with darker skin are needed
Electrolysis	Salon	Moderate	Long/ infrequent	Moderate	Yes	Find a certified electrologist
Chemical depilatories	Home	Low	Short/ infrequent	High	No	Not recommended for people living with cancer
Waxing	Home or salon	Low	Short/ infrequent	High	No	Not recommended for people living with cancer
Finasteride	Home	Moderate	Short/frequent	No	No	Not proven in people living with cancer; may only work when increased hair is hormone-related

will be less bothered by facial hair. When using eflornithine, hair removal (shaving, plucking, lasers, etc.) should also continue, as the cream will only reduce the frequency at which the hair needs to be removed. It should also be noted that the slowing of hair growth will only last as long as the cream is being used and that its cost will not be covered by insurance companies. Eflornithine can be used by women of any skin color or hair type. Most people are happy with the way it works.

Some people taking the targeted therapies cetuximab, erlotinib, gefitinib, or panitumumab may grow longer, thicker eyelashes and eyebrows. Some women say they like having more luxurious and curlier eyelashes, but it's important to see an ophthalmologist who can check your eyes and remove any ingrown eyelashes that could affect your vision. You could also carefully trim long eyelashes at home, using a small pair of scissors and a magnifying mirror.

> **DID YOU KNOW?**
> Hair gets its color from the pigment melanin, which is embedded into the strands when they are being formed. Dark hair has a lot of melanin, blonde hair has less, and gray hair has little to none; red hair has a different type of melanin altogether.

Hormonal Medications That May Cause Hair Thinning

Anastrozole

Bicalutamide

Estradiol

Exemestane

Fluoxymesterone*

Letrozole

Leuprolide*

Medroxyprogesterone*

Megestrol*

Nilutamide

Octreotide

Tamoxifen*

*Also may cause increased hair growth on the face

Anti-Cancer Medicines That May Change Hair Color

Lightening (to white or gray)	Darkening
Dasatinib	Cetuximab
Imatinib	Erlotinib
Interferon	Gefitinib
Ipilimumab	Panitumumab
Pazopanib	
Sunitinib	

Radiation Treatment and Hair Loss

About two to three weeks after beginning radiation therapy, hair loss may occur. But unlike chemotherapy, which can cause hair loss all over the body, radiation will cause hair loss only in the area that has been treated. So if radiation is given to a specific spot on the head, for example, that is where hair loss would occur. With radiation, hair loss also happens rapidly, with clumps of hair falling out in a short period.

The amount of hair loss depends on the dose and method of radiation treatment. For the most part, hair loss from radiation is pronounced if it is given to the brain. When very high doses of radiation are used, the hair in the treated area may be persistently thin or lost.

Q I'm starting brain radiation therapy next week. My friend who had chemotherapy recommended I cut off all my hair before it falls out. Should I do this?

A Radiation, which is often aimed at one spot on the head or body, does not have the same effect on hair as chemotherapy, which affects the entire body. If radiation is only aimed at certain parts of the brain, it will cause hair to fall out only in those areas. Since they may be only localized areas (unless whole-brain radiation therapy is being used), they can be covered with a different hairstyle or hairpiece. The best thing to do is to leave your hair as it is, so that longer strands of hair can be used to cover the areas with thin or no hair.

If no hair has grown after one year from the end of radiation therapy, the hair loss is likely to persist. For people who have already experienced hair loss from chemotherapy, persistent hair loss from radiation is more likely, since the hair has not been able to "recover." This is especially true if the chemotherapy included carboplatin, cisplatin, chlorambucil, cyclophosphamide, mechlorethamine, or oxaliplatin.

> **DID YOU KNOW?**
> Hair is made of a strong protein called keratin, the same kind of protein that forms the nails and the outer layer of the skin.

Persistent hair loss from radiation has been observed in children receiving radiation to the head for leukemia. High doses of radiation can cause inflammation of the skin (in this case the scalp), which later forms scars that harden (known as fibrosis), and hair follicles may be lost. Talk with your radiation oncologist about the dose and type of radiation you will receive, so you know what to expect. With low doses of radiation, and few cycles (or sessions), you can expect temporary hair loss. Remember, hair starts to grow back gradually, two to three months after treatment has ended.

Preventing and Coping With Hair Loss

There are ways to cope with hair loss, although there is no sure-fire way to prevent hair from falling out during treatment. However, some techniques, discussed here, work to a certain extent. Perhaps the best advice is to

 Q I'm getting a new type of chemotherapy (so-called targeted therapy), which is supposed to cause less hair loss. What should I expect?

 A There is very little hair loss when using the treatments known as "targeted therapies." Drugs such as cetuximab, erlotinib, gefitinib, panitumumab, sorafenib, and vemurafenib can lead to hair thinning (not complete loss) in about 30 percent of people. The hair tends to thin out about three to six months after starting treatment. After that, the hair tends to grow back, even while still on the medicine. Also, these treatments often cause hair to become curly or wavy, a look that many people say they like.

prepare yourself and try to limit the frustration about your new, but likely temporary, appearance. This may make the transition a bit easier for you and your family.

Various cosmetic options, such as wigs, hats, scarves, and turbans, have helped many people cope with hair loss (see page 113). Some people prefer to cut their hair shorter before treatment. With this approach, there is a less dramatic change in appearance. Still others find that shaving their head completely works best. It allows them to take control and make a preemptive strike rather than wait for their hair to fall out. Deciding among these options is strictly a personal choice. Whichever one feels right to you, both physically and psychologically, is the way to go.

When it comes to hair care products, choose mild shampoos and soft hairbrushes. Avoid hot rollers and curling irons when receiving chemotherapy. Using a soft or satin pillowcase reduces friction between the hair and scalp and can be more comfortable. Once hair is lost, be careful when going outside on a sunny day, as your scalp will be very sensitive to the sun. To avoid sunburn, you should apply sunscreen and cover your scalp with a sun-protective hat (see Chapter 10, "Sun Safety").

Ask your health care team about some of the treatments available to reduce the amount of hair loss. They include cold caps (also called scalp hypothermia), minoxidil (Rogaine) for the scalp and eyebrows, and bimatoprost for the eyelashes. Although none has proved to be 100 percent effective, you may find that some of these treatments work for you.

Cold Caps

Cold caps, ice packs, or similar devices placed on the head during a chemotherapy infusion work to lower the temperature of the scalp and reduce the flow of blood. As a result, smaller amounts of the chemotherapy reach the hair follicles, so the hair is less likely to fall out. Studies have shown that scalp hypothermia helps reduce complete hair loss in 50 percent of people, but the technique does not work for everyone.

Hair Apparent: Using a Wig, Hat, Scarf, or Turban

Most people feel better when they can cover their hair loss. A wig offers them a full head of hair, and possibly even a new look to feel good about. Some insurance companies will cover the cost of up to three wigs per year if your oncologist writes a prescription for a "full cranial prosthesis" (another name for a wig). Your oncologist can refer you to neighboring wig retailers. Wigs can be made especially for you or bought "off the rack." Work with a wig expert and try different styles of wigs before you buy one. The following sources offer more information about wigs and related products.

American Cancer Society www.cancer.org (877) 227-1596	Cancer Care www.cancercare.org (800) 813-HOPE (4673)
ACS Tender Loving Care www.tlcdirect.org (800) 850-9445	Tiffany Wigs www.tiffanywigs.com (800) 427-WIGS (9447)
Where There's A Need www.wheretheresaneed.org (866) 803-6095	Your HAIRx www.yourhairx.com (800) 374-4424
Wigging Out www.wiggingout.com (502) 418-8310	Wigs by Patti's Pearls www.wigsbypattispearls.com (800) 670-3292
Headcovers Unlimited www.headcovers.com (800) 264-HATS (4287)	Vogue Wigs www.voguewigs.com (888) 727-9447
Wigs.com www.wigs.com (800) 581-2001	Wigs For Cancer Patients NYC www.wigsforcancerpatientsnyc.com (212) 717-4000
Crickett's Answer For Cancer crickettsanswer.startlogic.com (717) 843-7903 or (301) 935-4411	Y-ME National Breast Cancer Organization www.y-me.org/programs/wig-prosthesis-bank.php (800) 221-2141
Cancer Fairy Godmother www.cancerfairygodmother.com	Heavenly Hats www.heavenlyhats.com (920) 264-7960
Halos of Hope www.halosofhope.org	Good Wishes Scarves www.goodwishesscarves.org

Doctors believe that scalp hypothermia may be effective only with chemotherapies that stay in the body for a short time, such as doxorubicin. People who receive chemotherapy daily or through a pump for several days would need to wear the cold cap most of the time, which is not practical. The cap is not useful for radiation-induced hair loss. Another concern with scalp hypothermia is the possibility that cancer cells could remain in the blood vessels in the scalp. Therefore, it may not be an ideal option for people being treated for head and neck cancers, leukemias, lymphomas, or in people who have metastatic cancer; or for those cancers that frequently spread to the skin, such as melanoma or breast, lung, ovarian, and colon/rectal cancers.

Finally, about 30 percent of people who use cold caps say that they feel uncomfortably cold and that the caps trigger headaches. Also, people for whom the cold caps did not work said that it made them feel worse about losing their hair. For these reasons, cold caps are not endorsed or used by leading oncology organizations and cancer centers. To find out whether scalp hypothermia is right for you, talk with your oncologist.

Minoxidil

This topical medication has been approved for use in men and women who have the type of hair loss that occurs with age. Although applying minoxidil to the scalp before and during chemotherapy may not prevent hair loss, it can reduce the amount of hair lost and speed up the regrowth of hair. One study in women with breast cancer found that applying minoxidil 2% twice daily on the scalp from the beginning of chemotherapy reduced by 50 days the amount of time it took for hair to start growing again. Women in this study applied minoxidil 2% twice daily from the first day of chemotherapy and up to four months after finishing treatment.

A 5% solution of minoxidil is now available, and although the product is labeled "for men," there is no reason why women can't use it. In men, the 5% formulation causes about 50 percent more hair to regrow than the 2% concentration. Although no studies have been conducted in chemotherapy-induced hair loss, the 5% strength, used twice daily, should be more effective

Hair Dyeing the Natural Way

Using hair dyes is something many women (and men) may want to do after chemotherapy (or during, if their treatment is the type that doesn't cause hair loss). Although it is safe to use hair dyes available at most salons, some people would prefer to use henna, a natural plant coloring made from the powdered leaves of a desert shrub plant, *Lawsonia inermis,* also called the mignonette tree. The American Cancer Society recommends the use of henna-based dyes for people who are concerned about the effects of chemical dyes. The following companies make henna-based natural products:

- Coastal Classic Creations
  www.coastalclassiccreations.com
- Pure Hearts & Clean Hands Soap Company
  www.phchnaturalsoap.com
- Aubrey Organics
  www.aubreyorganics.com
- Light Mountain Natural Hair Color & Conditioner
  www.light-mountain-hair-color.com/where.php
- Morrocco Method Int'l Henna
  www.morroccomethod.com

What you will need to dye your hair with henna:
- Henna dye (above-the-shoulder-length hair requires 4 oz [100 grams], longer hair requires twice as much)
- Hot water (be careful that it is not too hot)
- Bowl and stirrer
- Shower cap and a towel
- Disposable latex or vinyl gloves

Instructions: Remember first to test the dye on a strand of your hair before using it on your entire head. Start by mixing the henna with enough hot water (almost 1½ cups of water per 100 grams of powder) until you get the consistency of yogurt. With your gloves on, apply the henna paste to your hair in sections, beginning on the back of your head, and working forward. Put on the shower cap and leave the henna mixture on for 30 minutes to three hours. Rinse the henna paste out with lukewarm water and do not shampoo for the next two days.

Styling the Natural Way

These hair-styling products have few to no chemicals:

Organic Excellence Alcohol Free Styling Spray
(www.organicexcellence.com)

Free & Clear Hairspray
(www.psico.com)

Magick Botanicals - Hair Styling Gel Fragrance Free
(www.magickbotanicals.com)

Real Purity Natural Hair Styling Gel
(www.realpurity.com)

Suncoat Sugar Styling Mousse, Hairspray, and Serum
(www.suncoatproducts.com)

Max Green Alchemy Scalp Rescue Sculpting Gel
(www.maxgreenalchemy.com)

than the 2% formulation. However, further studies are needed to learn whether this form of minoxidil is a better way to manage hair loss or growth in people living with cancer.

Minoxidil is available as a liquid or foam (like a mousse). If there is no hair on the scalp, the liquid solution is easy to apply, but if there is still some hair, the

Q My treatment with docetaxel ended two years ago, but my hair has still not grown back fully. I was told there is nothing that can be done. What would you do for someone like me?

A The first thing I would do is to make sure that there is no other cause for your persistent hair loss. After examining the scalp to rule out other conditions and taking photos to document progress on subsequent follow-ups, I would check your levels of thyroid hormone (called TSH), vitamin D, and ferritin through a simple blood test. To get those hair follicles going, I would recommend minoxidil 5% twice a day, as well as oral supplements of biotin (2.5 mg or 2,500 mcg a day) and orthosilicic acid 10 mg a day (1 capsule twice daily).

I've decided I will be using minoxidil during my treatment to speed up hair regrowth. How long should I use it? Will my hair start falling out when I stop?

A study showed that minoxidil helped people who started using it from the beginning of chemotherapy up until four months after treatment ended. The ability to grow hair should be back to normal three to four months after finishing chemotherapy, so it is likely that minoxidil is no longer needed after that and hair will not fall out.

foam may be more convenient: it dissolves on the scalp as soon as it is applied. Remember, it is meant to go on the scalp, not the hair itself. Foams should be applied on a dry scalp.

Side effects of minoxidil include skin irritation, itching, and, in some cases, increased growth of fine hairs on the face. One in 200 women taking minoxidil develops increased facial hair. It must be noted that this is reversible, once use of minoxidil is stopped, and these fine hairs are usually easy to remove if they are bothersome.

Natural Shampoos and Conditioners

Vinegar Add two tablespoons of apple cider vinegar to a cup of water and apply it in the shower. Rinse.

Baking soda Add a tablespoon of baking soda to a cup of water and apply it in the shower. Rinse with lots of water. Be careful not to get it in your eyes.

Dry shampoo Use Oscar Blandi Pronto Dry Shampoo if you don't want to get your hair wet.

Natural brands Burt's Bees (www.burtsbees.com), Yes To Carrots (www.yestocarrots.com), e-sen-cia (www.e-sen-cia.com), Avalon Organics (www.avalonorganics.com), Aubrey Organics (www.aubreyorganics.com). Free & Clear (www.psico.com), Shikai (www.shikai.com), Dr. Hauschka (www.drhauschka.com), Max Green Alchemy (www.maxgreenalchemy.com), and Logona (www.logona.com).

Thin or Lost Eyebrows

Although chemotherapy can lead to loss of the eyebrows, they tend to look normal again after only a couple of months, since the hair is shorter. If the eyebrows have not regrown fully or are still thin three to six months after finishing chemotherapy, it's a good idea to consult a dermatologist. Your dermatologist will check for other causes of eyebow loss, such as low thyroid gland function, infections, autoimmune diseases, and, very rarely, certain types of cancer.

There are things you can do to make eyebrows fuller and thicker. Using an eyebrow pencil to create fuller eyebrows is a good way to start. The pencil color should match your hair (or wig color), being a bit darker. Use a light brown color if blonde, honey brown if redhead, and dark brown or black for brown or black hair.

Also make sure the shape of the brow brings out your eyes; create soft brows for small eyes. If your eyebrows are thin but still have some hair, brush the brows up and out across the arch. Then set the hairs with a product to keep them in place and pencil in missing areas. If there is no hair, use a powder to create your eyebrows. Stencils or eyebrow wigs are also good options.

Raise Your Eyebrows

The following products help regain your eyebrows. They can be obtained at Sephora stores or online at www.sephora.com and at www.eyebrowz.com:

Benefit Brow Zings Brow Shaping Kit

Smashbox Brow Tech To Go Pencil and Gel

SEPHORA COLLECTION Arch It Brow Kit

Too Faced Brow Envy Brow Shaping & Defining Kit

LORAC Take A Brow

Anastasia Beauty Express For Brows and Eyes

Eyebrowz Products (kits and eyebrow wigs)

Hiding, Not Seeking: On the Use of Camouflaging Products

Most of the time, people who experience hair loss or thinning are the first to notice it. But generally, other people are not aware of it until at least 50 percent of the hair is gone. There are many products that conceal areas in which the hair has thinned, and they are available in different colors (gray, blonde, brown, black, and many others):

- Hair thickeners (diCesare Thicken Hair Builder, Toppik Hair Building Fibers, proTHIK)
- Sprays and powders that cover the scalp (Top Coverage for Bald Spot and Thinning Hair, DermMatch Topical Shading, Bumble and Bumble Hair Powder, Fullmore Hair Thickening Spray)
- Masking lotions (COUVRe)

Eyelash Loss

Eyelash loss is a common side effect of chemotherapy, although it is rarely talked about. It tends to occur after hair on the scalp is lost. Besides the psychological effect of eyelash loss (also called madarosis), eye injuries and decreased vision can occur as a result of the lack of protection by the eyelashes during chemotherapy. Each upper eyelid has about 100 to 150 eyelashes; the lower lids have about half as many lashes.

There are several ways to deal with eyelash loss. False eyelashes can be used at any point during treatment. However, some people think they look unnatural. Another option is to have eyelash extensions, in which single lashes are glued to the eyelids. This procedure takes several hours, is expensive, and some people are allergic to the glue that is used.

Applying bimatoprost on the upper eyelid daily has been shown to make eyelashes thicker, longer, and darker in 80 percent of people not living with cancer, when used for at least four months. In addition, studies with bimatoprost in people living with cancer showed that after three months, the eyelashes were

Q

My chemotherapy is over, and my eyelashes haven't grown back very much. I want to start using bimatoprost. Can I apply it to the lower eyelid as well?

A

So far, bimatoprost has been tested only on the upper eyelid. In clinical studies, it resulted in thicker, longer, and darker eyelashes of both upper and lower eyelids.

three times longer and thicker and twice as dark. Doctors first noticed serendipitously that this medication caused eyelash growth in people with the eye disease glaucoma. Bimatoprost is available by prescription for the purpose of eyelash growth, but it is not covered by most insurance plans. It comes in a container with applicators to apply the solution at the root of the upper eyelashes only, every day for at least four months. Contact lenses and eye makeup should be removed prior to daily application of bimatoprost.

Eyelashes will remain longer and thicker for at least for one month after stopping the use of bimatoprost. It is not known whether lashes will remain thicker and longer for more than a month after stopping the medication. People who have used bimatoprost said they felt better about their looks and eyelashes.

Although bimatoprost is safe, it may cause some side effects. One in 20 people experienced infection, itching, irritation, redness of the eyelid (which is reversible when use of the drug is stopped) or permanent brown darkening of the iris (the round, colored area of the eye) and the eyelid. Although darkening of the iris is rare, it has been reported by some people and could be a concern to those with light-colored eyes.

There are many cosmetics that promise to grow longer, fuller lashes, none of which has been carefully studied for effectiveness or safety, so be careful when it comes to over-the-counter products. Although cosmetics may enhance the appearance of the eyelashes, they're unlikely to lead to eyelash growth. If you are missing eyelashes, it is difficult to use mascara, as it can get makeup in your eyes. So be aware of these factors before you spend a lot of money on these cosmetics.

There's Always Something That Can Be Done

For people with persistent hair loss that cannot be explained by any other disease, or that has not improved with minoxidil, biotin, or orthosilicic acid, hair grafting may be an option. Hair transplants can be done using a microscope and the follicular unit grafting technique. In this method, hairs are harvested from one part of the head and implanted on to another. Of course, to do this, there must be some hair in some areas of the scalp. The procedure is expensive, complicated, and time-consuming, but the new hair lasts for a long time and no longer thins.

The eyebrows can also be treated in this way, using either a strip of hair from the scalp (a transplant) when there is complete eyebrow loss or a few hairs at a time when eyebrows are thin. Eyelashes can also be transplanted, using hairs from either the scalp or the eyebrows. These procedures usually take one to three hours, must be repeated two to three times, and are usually done under local anesthesia in a doctor's office. Make sure you find a doctor who is trained to do this procedure. Consult the International Society of Hair Restoration Surgery (www.ishrs.org) or Hair Transplant Medical (www.hairtransplantmedical.com).

Preparing Yourself

There are several key steps to take, ideally before receiving chemotherapy or radiation therapy: understand the degree of hair loss usually caused by the treatments; decide whether to use medications to speed up hair regrowth (minoxidil for the scalp and bimatoprost for the eyelashes); consider various coverups (scarves, hats, turbans, wigs); and realize that in most people, hair loss is temporary. All of these steps will empower you and help you feel better about your appearance during treatment.

THINGS TO REMEMBER

- The loss of hair is usually temporary; hair will grow back within several months of finishing chemotherapy or radiation therapy.

- Hair loss from chemotherapy can occur throughout the body, including the head, face (including eyebrows and eyelashes), arms, legs, underarms, and pubic area. Radiation only affects hair in the specific area treated.

- Hair that grows back after chemotherapy may be different in color or texture but usually returns to its original look and feel within a few years.

- Various cosmetic options, such as wigs, hats, scarves, turbans, powders, and sprays, have helped many people with cancer cope with the loss of their hair.

- Cold caps and minoxidil may reduce the amount of hair lost from chemotherapy, although neither has proved to be absolutely effective.

- Bimatoprost is a good option to stimulate the growth and thickness of eyelashes.

- For increased hair on the face, threading, shaving, electrolysis, or laser removal are good options. Consider the best one for you based on cost, time it takes, and availability in your area.

- For greater hair and nail strength and growth, take the following supplements: biotin (2.5 mg [or 2,500 mcg] a day) and orthosilicic acid (10 mg a day).

- In cases where hair loss is persistent and cannot be explained by other causes, your doctor can check your blood levels of thyroid-stimulating hormone (or TSH), vitamin D, and the iron-storing protein called ferritin. Consider hair grafting or transplants as an option if nothing else has worked.

CHAPTER 7

Side Effects of Radiation Therapy

Radiation therapy is an effective way to treat many different types of cancer and to relieve symptoms, such as pain or growths. This treatment is often given for four or five days a week for five to seven weeks, although it can vary. Radiation destroys as many cancer cells as possible while limiting harm to nearby healthy cells. The dose of therapeutic radiation is many times greater than that used for diagnostic x-rays or CT scans.

In this chapter, you'll learn how radiation affects the skin, hair, and nails; what to expect (and when to expect it); medications your doctor can prescribe to treat side effects; and practical ways you can cope with symptoms. We'll start with an overview about radiation treatment and some of the advances that have made it such a sophisticated therapy.

Radiation can come from a machine outside the body (external-beam radiation therapy), which is the most commonly used technique. Radioactive material can also be placed inside the body, near cancer cells. This internal radiation treatment is known as brachytherapy. In a third technique, doctors sometimes use a radioactive substance given by mouth or into a vein. The substance travels in the blood to tissues throughout the body. Most side effects to the skin, hair, and nails, however, are caused by external-beam radiation therapy.

DID YOU KNOW?

Everyone is exposed to small amounts of radiation from natural sources every day.

The type of radiation treatment used will depend on many factors, including:

- The type of cancer
- The size of the cancer
- The cancer's location in the body
- How close the tumor is to healthy tissues
- How deep into the body radiation needs to go
- A person's age, health, and medical history
- Whether other anti-cancer treatments will be used

Advances in technology have made radiation treatment more effective. For example:

Three-dimensional conformal radiation therapy (3D-CRT) is one of the most common types of external-beam treatments. It shapes the radiation beam to the size and three-dimensional contours of the tumor and uses computers to plan and deliver the treatment.

Intensity-modulated radiation therapy, or IMRT, also conforms to the shape of the tumor. This technique modulates, or controls, very thin beams of radiation at varying intensities, and from various angles, for a custom-tailored radiation dose. IMRT is more costly and time consuming than other types of radiation treatments. However, some studies have shown that it can reduce skin peeling and pain by up to one third and also reduces mouth dryness (when used in head and neck cancer), thereby improving quality of life. At present, this technique is most often used to treat breast, prostate, lung, head and neck, and brain tumors.

Proton (or particle) beam therapy also delivers more precise radiation to tumors, sparing normal tissues from damage. Proton beam radiation is used to treat cancers of the eyes, brain, prostate, spinal cord, and soft tissue (sarcomas). At present, this type of radiation treatment is only available in about 30 centers worldwide, due to its high cost.

In general, radiation therapy may be used alone or in combination with other treatments, usually surgery or chemotherapy. For instance, many men who have cancer of the prostate receive only radiation therapy, whereas many women with breast cancer receive radiation therapy after chemotherapy and surgery, and those with head and neck cancers will have surgery first, followed by chemotherapy at the same time as radiation therapy.

Radiation can be given before, during, or after anti-cancer medications (chemotherapy or targeted therapies). Although using radiation and anti-cancer medications at the same time is more effective against many cancers, it also results in more side effects, such as radiation skin burns, mouth sores, or hair loss.

Because receiving chemotherapy or targeted therapies during radiation therapy increases the risk of developing a severe skin reaction or mouth sores, every effort must be taken to prevent these side effects and reduce their severity. If radiation is part of your treatment, talk with your health care team about your chances of developing side effects and the best ways to prevent and manage them.

Most people who receive radiation therapy can finish their treatment without major difficulties. The chance of developing side effects differs from person to person, depending on the sensitivity to radiation, also called radiosensitivity. The total dose of radiation received, how often it is delivered, and where in the body it is directed all play an important part in whether a person develops side effects from treatment. Although the side effects of radiation can build gradually over time, it's important to remember that most symptoms go away several weeks after finishing treatment.

How Radiation Affects Skin, Hair, and Nails

Early skin irritation (called acute radiation dermatitis) occurs in up to 80% of people with certain types of cancer at about two weeks after starting treatment and peaks four to six weeks later. Radiation dermatitis may last for two to six weeks after completing therapy.

DID YOU KNOW?

Between 50 percent to 60 percent of all people living with cancer will require radiation treatment as part of their care.

Symptoms include:

- Itching or pain
- Irritation in which the skin becomes swollen, red, and dry, like a sunburn; it may peel, crust, blister, or ooze fluid.
- Hair loss early on during treatment and lasting several months

As part of your radiation therapy, your doctor may prescribe topical corticosteroids—mometasone or betamethasone. These topical medications help prevent and reduce the symptoms of itch, swelling, pain, and inflammation from radiation. It is applied as a thin layer onto the skin once a day, from the day radiation begins to the day it is finished. Although there is virtually no corticosteroid absorbed into the body, and no concern about systemic side effects, less than one third of people receive preventive treatment for radiation burns.

It's important to note that these creams should not be used on open sores or in areas that are moist or draining. For open sores, topical antibiotics such as silver sulfadiazine, Polysporin, or mupirocin are effective in reducing harmful bacteria, which can contribute to inflammation and pain. In areas of moist desquamation (peeling), special dressings called hydrocolloids prevent infection and help the area heal faster. These

Q **Is there anything that puts me at higher risk for severe radiation skin irritation (dermatitis)?**

A Some factors can lead to more severe reactions: not washing the area with soap and water, weight and large breasts (women with breast cancer weighing more than 165 pounds or with a bra cup size D or larger), smoking, older age, infection of a surgical wound in the area, the use of chemotherapy at the same time, and underlying diseases such as diabetes or heart conditions. Cancers of the head and neck, rectum and anus, genitals, or breasts are more often associated with radiation-induced skin problems than other types of cancer.

Q For the past four weeks, I've been receiving radiation to treat my breast cancer. How do I know if the skin in that area has become infected and what should I do?

A Tell-tale signs of a skin infection include redness, swelling, pain, blistering, or peeling of the skin with a moist sore. This reaction, called "moist desquamation," occurs more often in the folds of the skin, such as in the armpits, under the breasts, near the genitals, and on the neck. If you experience moist skin peeling, talk with your doctor or nurse right away. They may obtain a skin culture and prescribe an antibiotic (such as cephalexin or trimethoprim-sulfamethoxazole).

bandages, which usually need to be changed daily, form a soft gel on the skin, covered with a special plastic that is water-, bacteria-, and oxygen-proof. The most commonly used hydrocolloid dressings are Comfeel, REPLICARE, 3M Tegasorb, and DuoDERM. Nurses with experience in wound care are your best allies when it comes to treating open sores.

When Radiation Is Combined With Anti-Cancer Medications: What You Should Know

By combining therapies, oncologists have found that they can treat cancer more effectively. This certainly seems to be true with radiation and anti-cancer medi-

Grading Acute Skin Irritation From Radiation

Severity	Characteristic
Grade 1 (mild)	Skin is pink, dry, or flaky
Grade 2 (moderate)	Skin is red, swollen, or has some open moist sores, especially in the armpits, under the breasts, or on the neck
Grade 3 (severe)	Skin has moist, open sores on flat areas; bleeding may occur spontaneously or from rubbing or scratching the skin

I was told to apply only a moisturizer (such as Aquaphor, Bag Balm, or one containing aloe vera) to the skin that will receive radiation, skin that will become very dry. Is there anything else I should do?

 Yes, there is definitely something better you can do, especially if you are treated with radiation for breast, head and neck, and genital cancers, since most people will experience pain, dryness, itching, and discomfort. The "dryness" is a consequence of the damage and inflammation, with subsequent peeling of dead skin cells that results from radiation. Consequently, treating the inflammation and the peeling skin is critical, and the only products that have been shown to help are moisturizers containing calendula and topical corticosteroids. These products should be applied during the entire treatment time, at least once daily on the area of skin receiving radiation.

DID YOU KNOW?

One study showed that in people with head and neck cancer who were treated with radiation, severe mucositis developed in 66 percent and increased to 98 percent when chemotherapy was given at the same time.

cations, particularly the new medicines known as targeted therapies (see Chapter 2, "All Rashes Are Not Created Equal," for more details on these new medicines). Combining radiation and either chemotherapy or targeted therapies usually does a better job of shrinking tumors than either treatment alone. These treatments are sometimes combined for cancers of the head and neck, esophagus, lungs, stomach, cervix, rectum, and anus.

Clinical studies have shown that about 85 percent of those who receive both radiation and the targeted treatment cetuximab, for head and neck cancer, may experience radiation dermatitis—which could be severe in almost 25 percent.

Because using radiation and anti-cancer medications together raises the chance of having more complicated side effects, it's important to be aware of the possibility. Talk to your doctor or nurse about preventive treatments or what to do if symptoms develop. Bringing the symptoms under control will enable you to continue benefitting from treatment and maintaining your quality of life.

Easing Skin Discomfort

Avoid prolonged exposure to the sun, which can further damage your skin. Avoiding direct sun exposure to the treated area is particularly important for people receiving radiation therapy. Radiated skin is also very sensitive to extreme weather, such as hot and sunny conditions. When you go outdoors, wear protective clothing and sunscreen. (See Chapter 10, "Sun Safety.")

Gently wash skin with soap and cool water and pat it dry to reduce skin irritation, redness, burning, itching, and moist peeling.

Take vitamins, but with caution. Antioxidants such as vitamin C or E protect healthy cells from damage, but they may also protect cancer cells. So before you take any vitamins, talk with your doctor first. He or she may advise you to use these supplements only after treatment has been completed. In general, only

During and After Radiation Treatment: Skin Care Tips

Wash the treated skin area with a gentle soap and lukewarm water. Avoid soaps or bubble baths that contain fragrance and do not use loofahs, scrubs, or sponges.

When using a towel, pat the area dry instead of rubbing it.

Wear loose-fitting, cotton clothing that does not rub the treated skin. For women, camisoles and loose shorts are less irritating to the skin when receiving breast or pelvic radiation.

Take short, cool showers or baths. Avoid hot water or prolonged immersion in water, which can dry your skin.

Your doctor may prescribe topical corticosteroids to reduce the swelling, redness, itching, and pain of early reactions (radiation dermatis) and to soften the skin in late reactions (skin fibrosis).

Topical or oral antibiotics may be used on open, sore areas of the skin with moist peeling, as they are often sites of bacterial infection.

If you would like to apply a moisturizer, you can do so after 15 minutes of applying the corticosteroid cream from your doctor. Some recommended moisturizers are Dove Cream Oil Shea Butter Body Lotion, Eucerin Calming Creme Daily Moisturizer, Vanicream Skin Cream, and Cetaphil Moisturizing Cream.

vitamin D, calcium, and a daily multi-vitamin are allowed, but this may vary. Ask your doctor whether your health care team works with an integrative medicine specialist who can discuss individual supplements. A good place to find out about herbs, botanicals, and supplements can be found at the Office of Dietary Supplements at the National Institutes of Health (www.ods.od.nih.gov) and at Memorial Sloan-Kettering Cancer Center (www.mskcc.org/aboutherbs).

Other Side Effects of Radiation Therapy

Mucositis (Sores in the Mouth, Genitals, or Anus)

Sores from radiation can be a serious problem because they can cause pain and infections, making it difficult to swallow, eat, drink, or use the toilet. Because the tongue, gums, and the tissues inside the mouth (the oral mucosa); genitals; and anus normally grow rapidly, they are susceptible to injury from radiation, which destroys cells that grow quickly. Mucositis usually appears one to three weeks after starting radiation. These types of sores can also affect the upper part of the throat and all parts of the digestive system. In cases where mucositis is expected to be severe, people may receive fluids and nutrition through a tube into the stomach or have a colostomy. About one third of all

Q **Which mouthwashes (and how much of each ingredient) have been shown to prevent oral mucositis, and how do I use them?**

A Swish two teaspoons (10 mL) of the mouthwash for two to five minutes four times a day and then spit out. An effective mouthwash should include a corticosteroid (dexamethasone 3.3 mg per 5 mL) and an antifungal (nystatin 500,000 USP units per 5 mL). If your doctor recommends Gelclair (protective coating), mix a packet with one to two tablespoons of water in a glass, stir and rinse the mouth for one minute, three times a day, one hour before meals.

people being treated for cancer develop mouth sores, especially those undergoing stem cell transplants, high doses of chemotherapy, or radiation to the anus, genitals, or head and neck. In general, mouth sores due to chemotherapy occur faster, at about 4 days after starting treatment. During radiation treatments to the head and neck, there are several techniques your radiation oncologist can use to decrease the incidence of mouth sores and even dry mouth. One technique is IMRT, explained on page 124.

The sores are often more severe when chemotherapy or targeted therapies are combined with radiation, occurring in up to 90 percent of people receiving radiation and chemotherapy. Secondary infections frequently occur, which may result in delays in chemotherapy or radiation therapy. These infections can sometimes become serious, especially if the immune system is compromised and white blood cells are at a low level. Make every effort to maintain your oral health with regular visits to your dentist. If your mouth develops sores from radiation, yeast may overgrow and cause an infection. If this happens, antifungal medications may be needed; antivirals may be required if a herpes infection appears.

There are a number of steps you can take to ease the discomfort of mouth problems:

- Use a soft toothbrush or sponge applicator to clean the teeth, gums, tongue, and soft tissue inside your mouth; this will help remove dried saliva, bacteria, and dead tissue.
- Choose soft foods that are easy to chew and swallow.
- Use a straw to drink liquids.
- Puree food in a blender or food processor.
- Avoid citrus fruits, coffee, alcohol, sharp foods (such as crackers or chips), as well as spicy foods.
- Rinse with an alcohol-free mouthwash (Biotene).

DID YOU KNOW?

Available outside the United States, the topical anti-inflammatory and analgesic benzydamine oral rinse (15 mL for 2 minutes, 4 to 8 times daily) is available. When used during radiation, it decreases sores and the need for pain medications.

- Use protective gels such as Oratect (with benzocaine) and Gelclair, which adhere to the inner part of the mouth. These medications form a coating that shields raw nerves.
- Use toothpaste for sensitive or dry mouth (Biotene, Sensodyne).
- Using medicated mouthwash mixtures frequently called "Magic Mouthwash" may be helpful. These mixtures contain a corticosteroid (dexamethasone), antibiotic (tetracycline), anesthetic (lidocaine), antihistamine (diphenhydramine), and antifungal (nystatin). However, they dampen the sense of taste, so many people dislike them.
- Use an alternative mouthwash, which I recommend to my patients: a solution with dexamethasone and nystatin to address the cause of the discomfort and provide long-lasting relief. Use it frequently and early on, when the mucositis is mild.
- In people with head and neck cancer, taking oral zinc sulfate (220 mg [50 mg elemental zinc]) three times a day during radiation therapy up until six weeks after will reduce the severity of mucositis.
- Pain control (with codeine-related tablets or patches) will be needed in most people.

Hair and Radiation

As discussed in Chapter 6, "Handling Hair Changes," two to three weeks after beginning radiation therapy, hair loss may occur. Hair will usually be lost just in the area that has received the radiation. After radiation therapy, hair loss may happen suddenly, with clumps of hair falling out very quickly. A recent study showed that persistent hair loss from radiation in pediatric cancer survivors is associated with anxiety and depression as adults. Therefore, any effort that may help to minimize this long-term effect is advisable.

Risk Factors for Persistent Hair Loss Due to Radiation

Hair already lost from chemotherapy when beginning radiation therapy

Prior chemotherapy with carboplatin, chlorambucil, cisplatin, cyclophosphamide, mechlorethamine, or oxaliplatin

Childhood leukemia treated with radiation therapy to the brain

Hair Care Tips During and After Radiation Therapy

Wash your scalp and hair daily with gentle shampoos and conditioners. Use Free & Clear or products that are sold as natural or chemical-free, including Avalon Organics, Blinc, Shikai Color Reflect, Dr. Hauschka, and Burt's Bees.

Do not cut or shave your hair. Leave your hair long, so you are able to cover areas of hair loss.

Try a wig, hair extensions, or hair thickeners (diCesare Thicken Hair Builder, DermMatch Topical Shading, or Toppik Hair Building Fibers) or sprays and powders that cover the scalp (Top Coverage for Bald Spot and Thinning Hair, Bumble and Bumble Hair Powder) until your hair gets back to normal.

Talk with your doctor when radiation therapy is completed about the possibility of using topical minoxidil 5% twice a day, oral supplements of biotin (Appearex 2.5 mg or 2,500 mcg a day) or orthosilicic acid 10 mg a day (BioSil, 1 capsule twice daily).

Although no hair growth one year after radiation therapy usually means that hair loss will persist, there is a possibility that some hair follicles are still alive and hair can grow from them. To determine this, a consultation with a dermatologist is advisable. The dermatologist may recommend a small skin biopsy. Many patients I treated over the years applied minoxidil (2% or 5% solution or foam) twice daily on the scalp, along with supplements of biotin (Appearex 2.5 mg or 2,500 mcg a day) and orthosilicic acid 10 mg a day (BioSil, 1 capsule twice daily). In some cases, hair growth was enhanced in previously bald spots. Remember that it takes a long

Q If I get brain radiation, can I still wash my hair with shampoo and conditioner?

A Thankfully, yes. There is no reason to avoid washing your hair (it will not make it fall out faster, as many people believe). In fact, using soap or shampoo on any area being radiated will keep it clean, reducing the chance of secondary infections and scalp irritation. Also, it is a good idea to leave your hair long, so you can comb over any areas of hair loss from the radiation should they appear.

time for minoxidil and supplements to work. Whenever hair loss is present, even with a history of radiation therapy, other causes such as low levels of thyroid hormone, vitamin D, or iron in the blood must be ruled out with a simple blood test.

Radiation Recall Dermatitis

It turns out that the skin appears to have a "memory." A condition called radiation recall dermatitis is one in which previously radiated skin becomes inflamed after a medication is given. Redness, swelling, itching, or skin pain (dermatitis) will appear after about one month of chemotherapy, targeted therapies, or antibiotics are given. This recall reaction can occur even if the skin did not become irritated when radiation was initially received. It is estimated that one in 20 people who receive chemotherapy after radiation therapy will develop this reaction.

Radiation recall dermatitis can occur from days to years after radiation therapy. This is seen more frequently with higher doses of radiation and certain chemotherapies, such as docetaxel, gemcitabine, and doxorubicin. This reaction must be taken seriously, because the mouth and internal organs can also experience recall inflammation. This reaction is probably a result of a continuous, low-level inflammation of the skin (and other tissues that may have been exposed) after radiation therapy, which is made more severe by chemotherapy or other medications.

Q I am receiving radiation for breast cancer. Can I wash the area with soap and use deodorant on my underarms?

A Washing the breast and underarm with soap and water every day has been shown to reduce skin irritation. It's fine to use deodorant, but avoid those that contain aluminum, as they can increase the amount of radiation to the skin. Examples of deodorants without aluminum are Tom's of Maine, Crystal Body Deodorant or Crystal Rock, Arm & Hammer Essentials Natural Deodorant, Adidas Cotton Tech Aluminum Free Deodorant, Desert Essence Dry by Nature Clear Deodorant Stick, or JĀSÖN Natural Products deodorant stick.

Topical corticosteroid creams such as mometasone or betamethasone will allow for continued administration of chemotherapy, since they effectively manage this symptom. Although corticosteroids are the mainstay of therapy, avoiding the sun, wearing loose cotton clothing, and using sunscreen can also help ease most of the discomfort.

Dry Mouth

Another complication from radiation, especially in people with cancers of the head and neck, is dry mouth, also called xerostomia. Dry mouth may also develop during radioactive iodine administration or chemotherapy and targeted therapies, but in these cases, it is either mild or temporary.

Dry mouth makes it difficult to eat or speak and allows the overgrowth of yeast and bacteria, which can result in thrush and cavities, respectively. Ask your doctor about new technologies that lead to less dry mouth, such as IMRT or the use of the medication amifostine, which prevents the damage of the salivary glands and minimizes dry mouth during and after radiation, and a surgical procedure that repositions the salivary glands.

Removing Radiation Tattoos

To aim the radiation beams precisely, radiation oncologists will tattoo tiny blue-black dots on the skin. The

Dry Mouth After Radiation: What Works

Method	Names	Efficacy/ Time of Effect
Gum	Biotene Dry Mouth Gum OMNI TheraGum Spry Chewing Gum XyliChew Gum Orbit Sugarfree Gum	Minimal/ brief duration
Lozenge	SalivaSure lozenges Numoisyn lozenges	Moderate/ brief duration
Gels or liquid	Biotene spray Optimoist Biotene Oral Balance Aquoral Artificial Saliva Mouth Kote Dry Mouth Spray Numoisyn Liquid	Moderate/ brief duration
Saliva stimulant	Cevimeline tablets Pilocarpine tablets	Good/ several hours
Acupuncture	On specific pressure points	Good/months to years

dots are made by placing a drop of dark ink on the skin and then using a sterile needle to permanently embed the ink in the skin. It can feel slightly uncomfortable, like a pinprick.

For people who object strongly to being tattooed because of religious or other reasons, a special type of pen can be used to draw a mark on the spot to be treated. The mark is then covered with a transparent adhesive dressing called 3M Tegaderm. Your radiation oncologist can tell you more about this option.

These tattoos are an important part of your treatment, and most of the time you are the only person who will notice them. But it's understandable that some people would like to have this reminder of their treatment removed once radiation is finished. There are two minor procedures that either a dermatologist or plastic surgeon can perform to remove the tattoos. They are both ambulatory procedures that are done in the office. The first is using a punch biopsy (essentially a small round blade), under local anesthesia to remove the tattooed skin (one stitch may be needed), to make the area heal better and faster. A tiny virtually invisible scar, the size of a pencil tip, may remain. The other technique involves using a laser to destroy the pigment in the skin. It takes about three sessions, spaced six weeks apart. Although both methods are equally effective, most people who have their tattoos removed prefer the laser because it doesn't leave a scar or change the skin color.

> **DID YOU KNOW?**
>
> Trolamine does not prevent or treat skin irritation from radiation. Equally ineffective are heavy, difficult-to-remove ointments such as Aquaphor, which some people can be allergic to because of the lanolin in it. Ask your doctor about topical corticosteroids that have been shown to work, such as mometasone or betamethasone.

Late Side Effects and Survivors' Skin

Although rare, skin reactions to radiation can occur as late as six months to 10 years after the end of treatment. Whether or not late side effects develop depends on the part of the body involved, radiation dose, length of treatment, other diseases such as diabetes, and whether more than one radiation technique is

Q I'm getting radiation to my pelvis for cervical cancer, with no chemotherapy. I suddenly developed this very itchy, red, bumpy rash on my trunk and arms. What is it, and what can I do about it?

A Skin side effects outside the area of radiation are very rare. However, an itchy, red rash can appear all over the body up to six months after radiation therapy. It has the unmemorable name of EPPER syndrome (for Eosinophilic, Polymorphic, and Pruritic Eruption associated with Radiotherapy). It usually occurs in women receiving radiation therapy for breast or cervical cancer. Treatment with topical corticosteroids will resolve it within a few days. Sometimes antihistamines like hydroxyzine or diphenhydramine can also be used to control itch.

used or chemotherapy or targeted therapies are also given. There is also some evidence to suggest that a genetic susceptibility or concurrent diseases such as diabetes, scleroderma, rheumatoid arthritis, or lupus may heighten the risk of tight, hard skin (fibrosis).

Late skin reactions include:

- Skin darkening
- Appearance of dilated, red blood vessels
- A tightness or hardness of the skin called fibrosis, which makes it difficult to move nearby joints
- Loss of hair, sweat, and oil glands
- Slow nail growth or nail loss if radiation is given close to the tips of the fingers or toes
- Wounds that don't heal, and scarring with inflammation
- Lymphedema in the skin or limb around the area
- Newly formed cancers, including skin cancer. It is important to be attentive to any growth in a radiated area, which should be examined and sampled by a doctor. They usually appear three years or more after radiation therapy.

I had radiation therapy for breast cancer three years ago, and the skin on my breast is very tight. My doctor said it's fibrosis. Is there anything I can do to make the skin softer?

Fibrosis is a typical late effect that develops in up to 30 percent of people treated with radiation for head and neck or breast cancer. In recent years, it has been shown that oral vitamin E and pentoxifylline can reduce the size of the fibrosis by up to 70 percent in two years. Taking 1,000 international units of vitamin E and 800 mg of pentoxifylline is recommended for at least three years. This treatment is more effective for those who received radiation therapy within the previous six years and for those also receiving physical therapy. Stopping this treatment early can cause the fibrosis to "rebound," so your doctor should carefully monitor your progress.

Since late effects from radiation affect so many people years after their initial diagnosis, treatment and ways to minimize these effects are described in Chapter 12, "Especially for Cancer Survivors."

Nail Changes After Radiation Therapy

Any part of the body can be affected by radiation, especially if it is in the path of the radiation beam. Fortunately for the nails, radiation to the hands and feet for cancers in those locations is relatively infrequent. Even total-body radiation therapy, as performed for Hodgkin lymphoma and other types of blood or lymph node cancers, does not usually affect the nails.

When radiation is aimed at a hand or foot, nail problems can include slower growth, brittle nails, dark discoloration, and loosening of the nails. Nail strengtheners such as Nail Tek can fill ridges (Nail Tek Foundation) and strengthen (Nail Tek II: Intensive Therapy for soft peeling nails and Nail Tek III: Protection Plus for dry brittle nails). Additional nail strengtheners that can be applied are OPI Nail Envy Nail Strengthener (Original), Sally Hansen Hard As Nails, and China Glaze Nail Strengthener & Growth Formula. If you decide to use nail polish, use a chemical-free brand such as OPI, China Glaze, Sally Hansen, Zoya, and Polished Mama. And don't forget to use natural nail polish removers such as Honeybee Gardens Odorless Nail Polish Remover, Suncoat Natural Nail Polish Remover, and Dr.'s REMEDY Non-Acetone Enriched Nail Polish Remover. Be sure to take at least 2.5 mg (2,500 mcg) of vitamin B_7 (biotin) every day, which makes nails grow faster and stronger.

All side effects of radiation, including late effects, should be reported to your health care team for assessment and treatment. This includes side effects unrelated to the skin such as memory loss, infertility, bone and joint changes, and low levels of thyroid hormone.

There are many ways to relieve discomfort and reduce the chances of further skin irritation. Most of these skin changes go away shortly after radiation

Q As a child, I had radiation therapy to my chest for lymphoma. I'm now 35, and since this was so long ago and I did not experience any skin reactions, is there anything to worry about?

A For survivors of childhood cancers, the risk of developing skin cancers is six times greater in areas that received radiation. Most of these skin cancers occur 15 to 20 years after the original cancer was diagnosed. Basal cell cancers, which are the most common and least dangerous, are the type usually found on the skin. More serious skin cancers are very rare. It's a good idea for all cancer survivors to be examined every year for any new or changing moles or spots on the skin, especially in areas of the body that received radiation.

DID YOU KNOW?

Some evidence suggests that the use of anti-estrogen drugs, such as tamoxifen, may make radiated skin tighter or harder. However, because these drugs are so important, they should continue to be used whenever prescribed.

therapy is over. However, in some people, skin that has been exposed to radiation might remain discolored and harder than it was before treatment and may be sensitive to sunlight.

The best way to deal with these side effects is to be prepared for them before they happen. Your health care team can offer you effective ways to prevent radiation-related problems from becoming serious. Take heart and remember that most of the side effects of radiation therapy go away shortly after treatment is over.

THINGS TO REMEMBER

- Radiation therapy that causes discomfort in one person may cause no side effects in another. Most skin problems caused by radiation are limited to the area being treated and go away within weeks after treatment is finished.

- Combining chemotherapy or targeted therapies with radiation therapy may cause more severe side effects than either treatment alone.

- It's recommended to wash the areas being treated with radiation with soap and water and to use deodorants without aluminum.

- Taking special care of your skin during radiation therapy is a must; topical steroid creams prescribed by your doctor may prevent the severity of reactions.

- Creams recommended by your doctor or nurse should be applied at least 4 hours before or after your radiotherapy session.

- Newer radiation therapy techniques (such as IMRT) have been shown to cause less skin irritation and less dry mouth than conventional methods, so ask your doctor about these methods.

- The mouth is frequently affected when radiation is given to the head and neck area. Controlling inflammation and infections, and later on dry mouth, is possible.

- Studies have shown that by preventing acute skin irritation, late effects (such as fibrosis) may be avoided.

- A physiatrist (doctor in physical medicine and rehabilitation) and physical therapist can help with skin tightness or hardness, pain, and neck deformities resulting from radiation therapy.

- Late skin problems after radiation therapy, such as persistent hair loss, dilated blood vessels, tattoos, and tight or hard skin, can all be improved with the help and guidance of a dermatologist experienced in treating cancer survivors.

CHAPTER 8

Your Skin After Surgery

Surgery offers the best chance of removing and curing many types of cancers. It can also be used to diagnose cancer (by obtaining a biopsy); relieve symptoms; and complement chemotherapy, targeted therapies, or radiation therapy.

DID YOU KNOW?

Surgery is the oldest form of cancer treatment; more than 1.5 million surgical procedures are performed every year for cancer.

In this chapter, you'll learn more about:

- The different types of surgeries and how procedures are performed
- Surgical wounds—how they heal and how to prevent complications
- Scars and how to prevent, reduce, and treat them
- Ports to administer chemotherapy and to draw blood
- Caring for pressure sores
- Skin problems in areas around a surgically created opening (stoma) made for the discharge of urine or stool.
- Lymphedema—its effect on skin and how to prevent and treat it

Surgical Cancer Treatments: From Older to Newer

There are several types of surgery for people with cancer, and each procedure has a different goal. *Curative surgery* removes the cancer; it's used when the tumor is located in a specific part of the body and has not spread. For instance, women with breast cancer may have the entire breast surgically removed (mastectomy) or only a portion of the breast containing the cancer (lumpectomy). People with lung cancer may have a part of a lung removed (lobectomy) or the entire lung removed (pneumonectomy). During curative surgery, the information learned by the doctor may help him or her predict whether the cancer is likely to return and whether additional treatment with anti-cancer medications or radiation is needed.

In *diagnostic surgery* (that is, a biopsy), a small piece of tissue is removed so it can be evaluated under a microscope. The results of this test can confirm a diagnosis, identify the type of cancer, or determine how far the cancer has advanced (the stage). Skin biopsies may also be performed by dermatologists to help diagnose rashes or skin cancers. For skin biopsies, procedures are done in the office, under local anesthesia, and take less than five minutes. Once your dermatologist has cleaned and sterilized the area, an anesthetic (usually lidocaine) is injected. This technique may be uncomfortable and may sting a bit. Then, a round device (called a punch biopsy) is inserted into the skin. A tiny piece of skin the size of a pencil eraser is removed and sent to the lab for analysis. A stitch (suture) is usually placed so that it heals better and faster. The stitch may be absorbable or may need to be removed two weeks later.

Doctors may also perform a lymph node biopsy or removal to find out whether the cancer has traveled to the lymph nodes. Lymph nodes are found in the neck, armpit, groin, deep in the stomach, and throughout the body.

Debulking surgery removes as much of a tumor as possible, often to make chemotherapy or radiation therapy more effective. This procedure is used when it's impossible to remove all of a tumor (possibly because doing so might harm an organ). Debulking surgery is also used to relieve the symptoms of cancer.

For instance, if a tumor is pressing on a nerve or bone, debulking surgery can relieve the pain and improve a person's quality of life. Although the cancer is not being treated in such cases, the symptom is being addressed, which is important in improving quality of life.

Preventive surgery removes tissues that do not contain cancer cells. If a person has a family history and/or a gene mutation that creates a very high risk of developing colon, breast, skin, or ovarian cancer, for example, preventive surgery may be recommended. Before they become cancerous, polyps in the colon, cysts in the breasts or ovaries, or moles from the skin may be removed.

Sometimes, surgery is the only cancer treatment needed. For example, women with certain types of gynecologic cancer (such as cancer of the uterus) may have a hysterectomy (surgery to remove the uterus) and do not require any further treatment. For a number of different cancers, from prostate to breast, surgery is used along with other treatments such as anti-cancer medications or radiation therapy. In such cases, surgery may come first. In other situations, chemotherapy may be given first, in the hope of shrinking the tumor before surgery. Tumors that are either too big or too difficult to remove with surgery may be better treated with other options.

Improvements in surgical techniques have led to less complicated and safer procedures. Because of these advances, patients may spend less time in the hospital, sometimes going home the same day as the procedure. For example, *cryosurgery* uses extremely cold liquid (such as liquid nitrogen, which is −321 °F) to freeze and destroy cancerous or precancerous cells. This approach has been used mainly in cancers of the skin and cervix, although it is being tested in other types, such as kidney cancer. *Laser surgery* uses beams of high-intensity light to remove very small cancers, shrink tumors, or activate drugs to kill cancer cells. *Radio frequency ablation* (RFA) is a procedure in which abnormal growths are destroyed using heat from a needle-like device placed inside the tumor that transmits a current. Interventional

DID YOU KNOW?

Wound healing is a complex process in which numerous cells are involved in clotting, inflammation, protein formation, and debris removal.

radiologists perform RFA procedures with the guidance of a CT scan or ultrasound. This technique is used to treat primarily liver, kidney, bone, lung, and pancreatic cancers. With *laparoscopic surgery*, a thin, tube-like instrument, called a laparoscope, is used to look at tissues and organs inside the body without the need for large incisions. The surgical methods described here aim to decrease the damage to healthy tissues by being "less invasive." This approach results in less scarring and faster recovery times.

What side effects you may experience after surgery depend on a number of factors: overall health, the type of surgery and cancer, and how advanced the cancer is. Most cancer operations cause some degree of pain or discomfort and a risk of bleeding and infection. In this chapter, the focus is on surgery and wound, scarring, and pressure sores. In most cases, these side effects can be managed with the help of your surgeon. In other cases, a dermatologist or plastic surgeon may be needed. Because infections are very rare and are usually managed with prescribed antibiotics or additional procedures done by your surgeon, they will not be discussed here. However, there are things you can do to improve scars and other issues relating to surgery; you'll learn more about them in the following pages.

Surgical Wounds: What to Expect

A cancer surgeon's objective is to gain access to a tumor in the body and either remove it or obtain a biopsy. But in doing so, the incision he or she makes creates a surgical wound—a physical injury that involves a break in the skin. Rest assured that the surgical team makes every effort to see that the surgical wound heals without becoming infected or painful and the appearance of the scar is the best possible.

The First Two to Four Weeks After Surgery

In the first month, the surgical wound is in its initial stages of healing. As the white blood cells remove any bacteria and damaged cells from the wound, there is considerable inflammation. During this time, blood vessels are forming to deliver nutrients to the wound. This inflammation and blood vessel formation can lead to some redness, swelling, and tenderness in the area, all of which are normal. Itching (what doctors call pruritus) is often part of the healing process of a surgical scar. In part, it is caused by stimulation of the nerve endings as they heal.

If you have itching with redness, blisters, or bumps around a scar, it may be caused by an allergy to antibiotic creams or ointments, tapes used to cover the wound, or even the solution used to wash the area before surgery (iodine-based or chlorhexidine). If you think you may be allergic to these products, one way to find out is by applying a small amount of the tape, cream, or ointment to an area without hair on the underside of your forearm and leave it on for one to two days, keeping it covered. If the area becomes red, itchy, or swollen, you are allergic to that substance and should avoid using it in the future.

If your surgical wound feels itchy, it's best to try not to scratch it, as this can lead to infections or more scarring. If an itchy rash appears around the surgical wound, be sure to tell your doctor. Oral antihistamines and topical corticosteroids can help ease this problem. (See Chapter 4, "How to Stop the Itching," for more information.) Apply the steroid cream to the inflamed, red area of skin, not in the actual wound, since this may delay healing. Make sure that your doctor is aware of your allergy and that it is noted in your medical records.

Normally, the skin on the edges of a surgical wound will close about 48 hours after surgery. In most cases, stitches, staples, tapes, or clips are placed to hold the wound together until it heals. Occasionally, a wound reopens or comes apart. Doctors call this problem dehiscence. When a wound opens, it may be simply a separation of the outer skin layers, but sometimes it involves deeper layers of skin and inner muscles.

DID YOU KNOW?

Surgical infections occur in five to ten percent of people who have surgery. Most people are given antibiotics before surgery, and sometimes during and after surgery, to prevent infections.

Many factors play a part in whether a wound heals properly. For instance, with surgery of the stomach and nearby organs, the age and gender of the person, type of disease, level of good nutrition, and long-time use of steroids may affect the skin's ability to heal. Smoking, diabetes, obesity, and rheumatoid arthritis also can slow the healing process. If you have a history of forming problem scars (keloids), and the procedure was done in an area that usually results in large scars (upper chest, back, arms, and ears), then your doctor may give you additional treatments immediately after surgery, such as corticosteroid injections or even radiation treatments.

Most surgical wounds heal without complications, but if a wound becomes infected, it's most likely to happen within the first month after surgery. Signs of infection include pain, swelling, redness, and oozing of yellow fluid from the wound. Two common types of wound infections are cellulitis and an abscess. Cellulitis, an infection of the deep tissues of the skin and muscle, may cause the skin to become warm and tender. An abscess, which is an enclosed collection of pus, usually causes a localized, round area of skin to become swollen and red. **If you see these signs of an infected surgical wound, alert your health care team immediately.**

Another complication after surgery is the formation of a hematoma, or blood collection, which can appear on the skin as a bruise in three to seven percent of people. Skin bruising or hematomas are more frequent in people living with cancer who are taking blood thinners for clots in the legs or the lungs. Hematomas can develop within days of the surgery, and they may need to be drained to prevent pain and infections in these pockets of blood that do not circulate.

There are several ways to successfully treat surgical wound complications:

- The wound may be opened, cleaned, and reclosed with new adhesive strips or sutures.

- When the problem is more severe, surgery to repair, drain, and reclose the wound may be performed.
- Some non-healing wounds may be treated with physical therapy using a whirlpool or warm bath.
- Antibiotics, which can be given orally, intravenously, or topically, are often prescribed to prevent or treat wound infections. It's important to finish all of the prescribed medication to make sure the infection is completely gone.
- Pain-relieving drugs such as acetaminophen, sometimes with codeine, are also helpful in dealing with wound pain. Avoid over-the-counter non-steroidal anti-inflammatories (such as ibuprofen or naproxen), unless prescribed by your doctor.

DID YOU KNOW?

About 1 of 200 women treated with surgery for breast cancer will develop redness of the breast, and the primary cause is infection.

The First Year After Surgery

In some cases, itching can last for months or even a year after surgery, as scar tissue continues to stretch. During this time, the scar is rearranging itself, laying down a tight weave of the strong protein collagen. During the first year, scars are only about 50 percent as strong as intact skin, and by the end of the first year, only about 80 percent as strong. Because scars never fully regain the strength of intact skin, it's important always to treat these areas gently.

Although surgical scars usually fade with time, they never completely disappear. For some people, the surgical scar may be small, easily hidden, and of little concern. For others, however, scars may be large and disfiguring, severely affecting their self-image. Because hair does not usually grow within a scar, disfigurement may be more noticeable on areas with hair, such as the scalp or a man's chest, arms, or legs. If you are having surgery on the scalp, leaving longer hair can help cover the scar.

Better Healing of Scars

If you have scars that have not healed, or have increased in size, it's important to tell your surgeon. Sometimes they could indicate the development of a hernia (out-pouching of internal organs), a newly formed skin cancer, or a recurrence of an underlying tumor.

There are several ways to reduce the size, pain, tightness, and appearance of a surgical scar. Sometimes a single treatment can significantly improve the look of a scar. In other cases, a combination of approaches may offer the best results. Consult with your doctor or a plastic surgeon to find the right treatment for you. Here are a number of side effects associated with scars and ways to mange them.

Itching Use topical corticosteroids as ointments, creams, or medicated adhesive tapes daily. Corticosteroid tapes form a barrier over the scar, which prevents irritation of the skin from scratching.

Redness or dilated blood vessels These color changes may last a long time and can extend beyond the scar, especially if the skin also received radiation. One year after the surgery, laser treatments at a dermatologist's or plastic surgeon's office will usually take care of this. Normally, several sessions are needed, and a slight stinging pain occurs when the laser is used.

Pain Corticosteroids can either be applied topically or injected by a dermatologist or plastic surgeon. Also, creams or patches containing numbing medicines such as benzocaine, lidocaine, or pramoxine can be used. A visit to a physical medicine and rehabilitation doctor or plastic surgeon may also be in order. They can recommend special physical therapy or perform a small surgical procedure on the scar to fix it (known as a scar revision).

Tightness Physical therapy is a great way to improve mobility of tight scars and joints. If this is ineffective, a plastic surgeon may have to operate and perform a scar revision.

How do I know whether I have an abnormal "problem scar" that could be improved?

 There are a few things to look for. It's a problem scar if it:

- Grows too much (called hypertrophic, keloidal)
- Is associated with pain or itching
- Is physically or psychologically unacceptable
- Restricts movement of joints or limbs

Problem scars occur in an estimated 10 percent of all wounds, and they appear most commonly on the upper back, chest, earlobes, and thighs. They are rarely found on the face, genitals, hands, or feet.

Large scars Aside from surgery, no method can make a large scar completely go away. Injecting corticosteroids or other chemotherapy medications into the scar may shrink it. If surgery is used, it can be followed by radiation or topical medications to prevent regrowth.

DID YOU KNOW?

It takes about one year after surgery for a scar to heal completely.

Darkening Bleaching creams, such as hydroquinone 4%, special peels, or lasers may be recommended by your dermatologist or plastic surgeon. Because sunlight and even light from indoor fluorescent bulbs will make skin darker, you always need to apply sunscreen over the scar.

Cutting Out Keloids

Keloids are large, abnormal scars. A keloid may be flesh-colored, red, or pink and may be lumpy or ridged. It may also itch while it is forming and growing.

If you have a keloid or problem scar, a plastic surgeon can align the incisions for a better appearance of the scar. This is done through a procedure called "scar revision." In this process, a plastic surgeon removes excess scar tissue and aligns the scar so that it is less noticeable. Depending on the size of the scar, it can be done either in the surgeon's office under local anesthesia or in the operating room.

Ways to Improve the Signs and Symptoms of a Problem Scar

Technique	What It Does
Silicone sheets and gels	They give moisture to scars, making them softer and less likely to grow. Silicone sheets have been shown to reduce the size of scars. The sheets and gels should be applied for at least 12 hours a day. Example sheets are Epi-Derm, ScarAway, Scar Fx, and Avogel. Examples of gels are Xeragel, Pro Sil, and Avosil.
Chemical peel	A peel is a chemical solution that causes a controlled destruction of a part of the skin; new, more flexible skin replaces the older, damaged skin. To be used with caution or avoided in people with dark skin, as well as those who are prone to form keloids, or those with an active skin infection.
Debridement	When there is an open wound and a scar has not properly formed, the removal of damaged or infected tissue allows normal skin to grow.
Dermabrasion	A rapidly rotating brush is used to "sand" the top layer of skin to improve its irregularities. The skin becomes smoother and rejuvenated as a new layer of remodeled skin replaces the older, damaged skin. Used for acne scars or excessive growth of skin in large areas.
Hyperbaric oxygen	High levels of oxygen promote healing in surgical wounds, ulcers that do not heal, and in previously radiated areas of skin.
Intralesional injection	A medication to shrink and soften problem scars is injected every four to six weeks (usually needs to be done three or four times). Medications used include a corticosteroid (triamcinolone), chemotherapy (fluorouracil, methotrexate, bleomycin, mitomycin C), or others (verapamil, botulinum toxin A).
Fillers	Collagen (a protein that supports the skin) or fat is injected into the skin to fill in dimpled scars. The surface of the scar is brought even with surrounding tissue. Results may last from a few months to several years.
Laser treatment	A concentrated beam of light is used to remove the outer layer of skin or blood vessels, allowing new, firmer, smoother skin to form. People with dark skin have to be careful, as laser treatments can change skin color.

Ways to Improve the Signs and Symptoms of a Problem Scar (cont'd)

Technique	What It Does
Negative pressure wound therapy	A suction device is used to manage abdominal wounds that will not heal. Whether this procedure really works is controversial.
Radiation treatment	Usually given shortly after surgery, in people with a history of problem scars, radiation can reduce or prevent excessive scar growth.
Topical medications	Medicines used to block collagen formation in the scar. Topical gels or creams include corticosteroids, anti-fibrosis (imiquimod), salicylic acid, and vitamin A (tretinoin 0.05% cream).
Surgery	Done by a plastic surgeon to remove excess scar tissue and make the scar less visible, this procedure is called "scar revision." Surgery on a scar should not be performed before the first year, as the scar is still forming.

Mastectomy and Expanders

After a mastectomy, to accommodate breast implants, temporary tissue expanders are placed in the chest to stretch the skin so there will be enough space for the implants. In about one third of women, the pressure exerted by these implants on the breast skin may impair flow of blood in the skin. This rarely leads to inflammation and the formation of red, scaly areas on the skin. Because the skin over this area usually does not have any sensation after surgery, there will be no pain or itching. Using a topical antibiotic (mupirocin) along with a corticosteroid cream (fluocinonide) twice daily for two to four weeks usually resolves this problem. If a breast rash or an area of red skin does not improve with these topical treatments, a skin biopsy is strongly advised to rule out a cancerous growth.

Ports and Complications

Ports provide ready access for the delivery of anti-cancer medications, fluids, antibiotics, transfusions, and nutrition. They eliminate the need for painful needle

I had my surgery last week. Is there anything I can do to prevent the formation of a problem scar?

Pressure and friction stimulate the cells that form scars, so it's best to avoid stretching or massaging the area. The stitches should be removed at the appropriate time—taken out too soon, the scar may widen; taken out too late, they can leave "track" marks. Apply the topical antibiotics or dressings recommended by your surgeon. Avoid exposing it to the sun; keep it covered, and use a sunscreen with an SPF of at least 15 for the first four months after surgery. Studies have shown that over-the-counter creams containing vitamin E or onion extract (such as Mederma) do not reduce the formation of scars.

DID YOU KNOW?

After a mastectomy, a tissue expander may be placed to make room for a permanent implant. Apply a small amount of a topical antibiotic (mupirocin) at the site every time after it is injected (or expanded).

sticks and repeated attempts to access a vein in the arm or hand.

Most ports are placed on the upper chest in a relatively simple procedure using local anesthesia. In three percent of people, this wound will not heal well. One out of six people can have port infections, especially younger people and those with a blood-related cancer, such as leukemia. Five percent of ports can become blocked (sometimes due to blood clots), and in less than one percent of people, the port can stick out from under the skin, mostly in people who are very thin.

Slightly more problems occur when ports are placed on the left side of the chest and in people who are overweight. In some cases, for example in ovarian cancer, or for fluid accumulating within the abdomen, ports are placed over the stomach. The scars from all ports tend to be small, and once the port has been removed, certain measures can be taken to improve the cosmetic appearance of the scar (See the box entitled "Ways to Improve the Signs and Symptoms of a Problem Scar" on page 152.)

A survey of 356 people living with cancer showed that more than 90 percent were very satisfied with their ports and would recommend them to someone in a similar situation. Most people even decided to keep

Q Will physical therapy help with scars? How do I know if I need it?

A Physical therapy can help if you experience any of these side effects as a result of surgery: a tight scar, pain, lymphedema, or tightness or weakness of the area or nearby limb. Tightness can be improved with the help of a physical therapist. Your doctor can determine whether you need physical therapy or an evaluation by a physical medicine and rehabilitation doctor.

the port after their treatment had been completed, in case they needed additional therapy. Once your port is removed, talk with your dermatologist or plastic surgeon about ways to improve the scar if you are not satisfied with the way it looks.

DID YOU KNOW?

Unlike what many people think, massaging scars will not prevent, soften, or make them look better.

Pressure Sores: How to Prevent and Treat Them

A pressure sore (also known as a bedsore) is another condition that may affect the skin after surgery, especially in people unable to move from a bed or chair for a long time. These open, crater-like skin sores (or ulcers) are caused by constant pressure or friction against the skin, resulting in decreased blood flow to the area; to stay healthy, tissues require continuous blood flow and the nourishment it delivers.

More than one million people develop pressure sores every year in the United States. People who are bed- or chair-bound, with very moist or dry skin, cardiovascular problems, poor nutrition, and advanced age are at higher risk. These sores can lead to pain, infections, fever, oozing fluid, and skin swelling. Although bedsores can occur on different parts of the body, the most common places are the heels, hips, ankles, and lower back (tailbone). A bedsore can result from just one long episode of staying in the same position, but it usually develops after repeated incidents of many days or months of friction or pressure in one area.

Most pressure sores can be prevented or treated. Prevention is key, since pressure sores can prolong the length of a hospital stay. Here are a few standard precautions used by most health care providers to prevent the occurrence of pressure sores or to heal existing ones.

Move your body around (reposition), when in bed, or sitting in a chair, to a different position every one to three hours. People who need help moving should be lifted, not dragged. Keep bed linens smooth and unwrinkled.

Use special high-specification foam mattresses to avoid constant pressure or friction. Pressure pillows, sheepskin, foam padding, and powders also help relieve pressure on the skin. For chairs, use pressure-redistributing seat cushions. On the other hand, donut- or ring-shaped cushions have not been shown to be helpful.

Observe the skin daily for redness and swelling, both of which are the early signs of a pressure sore. Always avoid pressure over the sore and positions that result in greater pressure over the area (semi-sitting, sitting up straight, slouching). On a bed, position should be flat or at a 30 degree angle, laying on the side; heels should be elevated.

Keep the skin dry. Sweating or incontinence increases the chances of pressure sores. Incontinence should be treated and undergarments changed regularly. After bathing, the skin should be thoroughly dried.

Avoid massaging the area. The area should be left alone so it has time to repair itself. Massage can aggravate bedsores. Instead, use a barrier cream that minimizes friction (zinc oxide 13%–40% cream).

Maintain proper nutrition. Eating healthfully and drinking plenty of water provide the skin with essential minerals for repair. A consult with a nutritionist may be advisable.

Treating a pressure sore depends on how deep it is and whether it's infected. Treatment options may include:

- Caring for the wound with protective dressings (Allevyn Adhesive or Sacrum,

Comfeel, DuoDERM are good examples);
dressings should be changed every two to
three days or longer to prevent irritating the
sore.

- Special suction devices (called negative
  pressure wound therapy)
- Whirlpool baths in a rehabilitation or
  physical therapy facility
- Oral and/or topical antibiotics, generally
  used if the pressure sore has signs of
  infection or odor. Pain medications to
  alleviate discomfort from the sores are also
  recommended.
- Requesting a visiting nurse is a good idea, to
  help with dressing changes and wound care
  at home

For severe pressure sores, surgery can be performed
to remove damaged skin or to replace it with healthy
skin from another part of the body (a skin graft). This is
usually done by a general or plastic surgeon.

Skin Problems Related to Ostomies
(Surgical Redirection of Urine or Stool)

In some cases of colon, rectal, or bladder cancer,
parts of the organ, or the entire organ, are surgically
removed. In order for the person to discharge body
wastes, the surgeon performs an ostomy, or an opening in the body. The stoma is the end of the urinary
tube or intestine, which can be seen coming out of
the abdomen. A special bag (also called a pouch) is
attached to the stoma to collect stool or urine. The bag
is usually changed every other day, depending on the
accumulation of waste. The bag adheres to the skin,
sometimes using a round appliance, or "wafer," made
of a flexible adhesive material. Bags can be one- or
two-piece systems, which collect waste and protect
the skin from infections and irritation.

Less than 50 percent of people with a stoma develop skin problems around the opening, and most issues

Stomas and Skin: What You Need to Know

More than one million people in the United States are living with stomas.

Skin side effects will appear in 48 percent of people with urinary diversions (ileal conduits); 57 percent of small intestine diversions (ileostomies); and 35 percent of large intestine, or colon, diversions (colostomies).

Complications in stomas can occur any time from the first month to years after surgery, so it is always important to be vigilant.

The wafer (connection between the stoma and the bag) can loosen if the stoma is in an area of friction (under the belt) or near dimpled skin.

Skin complications include irritation, itching, sores, infections, hernias, tissue growths, and allergies to any of the materials of the appliance.

Skin irritation and rashes around the stoma can occur from urine, feces, or the pouch products used.

Stoma nurses can help reduce complications, so follow-up visits are recommended two to four weeks after the surgery, three and six months later, and then every year for the rest of a person's life.

DID YOU KNOW?

Allergies in people with stomas may be the cause of a rash, with the adhesive paste being one of the most common culprits.

appear after the first month. Most people don't realize that they're having a skin problem, and few seek help for it, so it's a good idea to keep appointments with your stoma nurse, who is extremely knowledgeable and helpful and will minimize and treat complications.

Weeks after surgery, irritation around the stoma can appear as redness or sores. This can be caused by urine or stool leaking, an incorrect location of the stoma, changing the appliance too frequently, incorrect removal of the adhesive wafer, or a pouch that is too large for the opening.

Years after surgery, skin growths and sores can occur in areas of chronic irritation around the stoma, which can bleed or hurt. This occurs more frequently in people who haven't seen a stoma nurse in a long time, when the appliance is too hard or ill-fitting, when the ostomy support belt loosens, or when the stoma opening is too large. Crusts around the stoma may also develop in one fourth of people who have the bladder

Stomas: What Should I Do if I Have...

Irritation

- Make sure the pouch is the right fit and size. Talk with your stoma nurse about changing your appliance if it is not easy to use or does not fit.
- Use a convex pouch. This type of pouch curves in toward the abdomen and is designed to improve wearing time, reduce leakage, and prevent irritation.
- Fill in skin creases with a thick paste or ointment recommmended by your stoma nurse.
- Use hydrocolloid powder on moist or broken skin, to provide a dry surface for the wafer.
- Use a corticosteroid (triamcinolone, clobetasol) spray at every change. For irritation from frequent changes, try to hold the skin during removal and pull in the direction of hair growth. Use a skin sealant to increase the time between changes.

Growths around the stoma

- Use a pouch system that covers the growths.
- Change the pouch every three days until the growths improve.
- Apply hydrocolloid powder and thick paste over the growth so that the wafer can be placed over it.
- Ask your doctor about silver nitrate chemical cauterization to treat the growth.
- An evaluation by your surgeon is important to rule out a hernia or a cancerous process.

Crusting

- Drink more water.
- Take 1 gram of vitamin C daily.
- Apply vinegar-and-water–soaked pads for 20 minutes at every pouch change.

Sores from pressure

- See your stoma nurse for resizing of the device.
- Select a flatter or softer pouching system.
- Loosen the ostomy support belt.

Stomas: What Should I Do if I Have... (cont'd)

Infections
- Your doctor may obtain a culture of the area to determine which germ is causing the infection and what antibiotics will destroy it.
- Antifungal (nystatin, miconazole [Zeasorb-AF], terbinafine [Lamisil AF Defense]) or antibacterial (Polysporin) powders should be applied at every change.
- Oral antifungal (fluconazole) or antibiotic (ciprofloxacin, levofloxacin, trimethoprim-sulfamethoxazole) tablets may be necessary.
- Dry the area after sweating.
- Remove hair with clippers or scissors; pull device in direction of hair growth.

Allergies
- Remove the product causing the allergy.
- Use corticosteroid sprays at every change (triamcinolone, clobetasol). These sprays dry quickly and will not interfere with using the appliance.
- If a cause cannot be found, see a dermatologist who will test your skin for allergies.

removed (ileal conduits). They result from urine deposits that have become solid and may bleed or hurt.

Skin infections can occur several months after a stoma is placed. People experience redness, pain, burning, pus, and bumps. Risk factors include excessive sweating, frequent leaks, shaving the area, or use of oral antibiotics. Skin allergies are common and are marked by itching, redness, rash, scaling, or even blisters near the wafer. These allergies may be caused by the pouch system or by soap and fragrances in skin products. When the area is irritated, burns, itches, or is painful, using topical corticosteroid sprays (clobetasol, triamcinolone) along with a topical antibiotic powder (Polysporin) will usually provide relief.

Lymphedema

If you have lymph nodes removed and/or radiation as part of your cancer treatment, you may be at risk for developing lymphedema. This condition is a swelling that happens when the body's lymphatic fluid cannot circulate properly and builds up in the soft tissues. Lymphedema usually develops in an arm or leg but can also occur in the hands, feet, or even the breasts. The condition is most often associated with breast cancer and the removal of lymph nodes from the underarm. But it can result from removal of lymph nodes in the groin during treatment of genital cancers, as well as melanoma, or cancers that have spread to the lower abdomen. Lymphedema can occur months to years after surgery and is more likely to happen in people who are overweight. It can significantly affect a person's quality of life and ability to perform daily activities.

Lymphedema also predisposes the skin to more frequent and serious infections. Most of these infections can be treated with oral antibiotics. However, every effort must be made to prevent lymphedema and such infections. Ways to prevent and treat lymphedema are presented in the box in the next page. Work closely with a lymphedema therapist early and throughout the entire process.

DID YOU KNOW?

Lymphedema affects women with breast cancer who undergo axillary (armpit) lymph node dissection (in 12 to 28 percent) or sentinel lymph node biopsy (in 4 to 8 percent).

Q When can I start using deodorant after my lymph node dissection?

A It's best to wait until the wound is completely healed, which is usually one month after surgery. Most doctors recommend that you use deodorants without aluminum such as Tom's of Maine; Crystal Body Deodorant, Crystal Rock, or any type of Crystal deodorant; Arm & Hammer Essentials Natural Deodorant; Adidas Cotton Tech Aluminum Free Deodorant, Fitness Fresh; Desert Essence Dry By Nature Clear Deodorant Stick; or JĀSÖN Natural Products Deodorant Stick.

How to Prevent and Treat Lymphedema

Lymphedema is a serious condition that should not be ignored. If left untreated, it can get worse and may cause more serious problems. But there are a number of steps you can take to avoid them:

Protect the area from trauma

- If the area needs to be shaved, use an electric razor.
- If an arm is affected, do not have shots, blood drawn, or your blood pressure taken on that side. Wear an alert bracelet on the affected arm.
- Avoid wearing tight clothing or jewelry on the area.
- Carrying heavy packages, luggage, or shoulder bags puts stress on your affected limb and could cause more swelling and pain.
- It's best to bring your own nail care supplies when having a manicure. Ask the manicurist not to cut your cuticles.
- Use sunscreen or protective clothing when going outside to avoid sunburns in the area.
- Treat scratches, cuts, and insect bites by cleaning the area and applying a topical antibiotic.
- If you notice swelling/redness, contact your doctor immediately.

Wear special garments

- A compression sleeve helps drain the lymph fluid.
- A doctor's order will ensure that you see a lymphedema therapist and obtain a custom-tailored sleeve, glove, or stocking that fits you.
- Gloves, stockings, and compression sleeves should be worn whenever doing activities such as gardening or during air travel.

Elevate, exercise, and massage

- The main goals of lymphedema therapy are to reduce the swelling and prevent infections and to maintain function of the area, arm, or leg.
- Whenever possible, keep the area elevated.
- A lymphedema specialist can teach you special exercises and perform a manual lymph drainage massage. This type of massage helps move the fluid from where it has settled. Afterward, the affected limb is wrapped in special padded bandages.
- All of these methods are best done under the guidance of a therapist recommended by your oncologist. For more information, contact the National Lymphedema Network at (800) 541-3259 or visit www.lymphnet.org.

Q What's the advantage of seeing a lymphedema therapist?

A This type of specialist will guide you through complete decongestive therapy, which includes skin care, compression garments, exercise, and manual lymph drainage. The therapist will also manually massage the affected area, to improve the flow of lymph fluid.

Summary

Most surgeries for the treatment of cancer will be uneventful. Surgeons and their teams take great care in preventing problems before they happen. However, in the rare case that something adverse may happen, knowing what to do will keep you a step ahead of significant complications. As always, do not wait to contact your doctor if you feel something is wrong—helping you feel better and improving your health are always the goals. Wounds, scars, ports, stomas, and lymphedema can all be cared for in a way that minimally affects your life so you can recover as quickly as possible.

DID YOU KNOW?

Maintaining an ideal body weight is critical to keeping lymphedema under control.

THINGS TO REMEMBER

- Surgery is an important part of most cancer treatments; there are doctors who specialize in the surgical treatment of cancer (surgical oncologists).

- Surgical complications are not very common, but when they do occur, there are many things you can do to resolve them.

- Most surgical wounds heal without complications within about two weeks after surgery, but the scar continues to repair itself for up to one year after surgery.

- Problem scars (those that are itchy or large) can be improved with topical or injectable medications, laser, surgery, or radiation.

- Most people who have a port placed in the chest for injections are satisfied, since it is easier to draw blood and to inject chemotherapy; the rate of complications with ports is very low.

- The best way to treat a pressure sore is to prevent it in the first place. Frequent movement of body position to relieve weight, along with special dressings and topical antibiotics, will help in most cases.

- Some anti-cancer medications (including bevacizumab, doxorubicin, fluorouracil, hydroxyurea, and sorafenib), as well as corticosteroids, may need to be stopped a few weeks before and after surgery, as they can prevent wounds from healing properly.

- Lymphedema occurs in many people who have lymph nodes biopsied, removed, or radiated. Using a compression garment and working with a lymphedema specialist are keys to maintaining normal function and preventing any complications.

- Rash or sores may develop around stomas; having the appropriate appliance, preventing leaks, and using corticosteroid sprays and antibiotic powders will usually resolve them.

CHAPTER 9

Stem Cell Transplants and Your Skin

One of the most exciting advances in the treatment of blood, bone marrow, and lymph node diseases and cancers is the use of stem cell transplants. With this technique, doctors can replace diseased blood cells—in a person with leukemia or lymphoma, for example—with blood-forming cells from a healthy person. By removing cells that are not working properly and giving healthy stem cells, transplant doctors aim to cure the condition and restore the healthy function of the blood cells.

The cells that are given in a transplant are called the "graft," the person who gives the cells is referred to as the "donor," and the person receiving them is the "host" or "recipient." Stem cells can be donated from a family member, a stranger, an infant's umbilical cord, or in some cases people themselves.

Because the body's immune system recognizes and rejects infectious organisms or tissues that are not its own, it's important that donated stem cells be as genetically close (or "matched") to the recipient as possible. To ensure this, transplant doctors carefully look for a genetic similarity between the donor and the recipient. Before the transplant, the recipient, or host, is given high doses of chemotherapy (known as ablative or myeloablative conditioning) and/or radiation (frequently in the form of total-body irradiation). This pre-treatment removes the patient's defective cells and "knocks out" his or her immune system to prevent re-

DID YOU KNOW?

For some types of disorders and cancers of the bone marrow, lymph nodes, and blood, transplants of healthy stem cells from bone marrow, blood, or umbilical cords provide the best option for a cure and the greatest possibility of remaining cancer-free.

Transplants, by the Numbers

The Center for International Blood and Marrow Transplant Research, which includes more than 500 transplant centers in 54 countries, reports that approximately 60,000 transplants were performed worldwide in 2009. In the United States, approximately 12,000 autologous and 5,000 allogeneic transplants were performed in 2009.

DID YOU KNOW?

Doctors do not recommend that transplant recipients receive the shingles vaccine, since there is no information on its safety. The chickenpox vaccine is optional and the human papillomavirus (HPV) vaccine should be given according to local guidelines.

jection of the donated cells (or graft). People who are older and/or those who have other health problems may not be able to tolerate the high doses of chemotherapy. For them, the transplant team may consider less intense chemotherapy (called nonmyeloablative or reduced-intensity conditioning). Reduced-intensity conditioning is also used for situations in which the risk of the disease reappearing later may not be as high, such as Hodgkin lymphoma, myeloma, and some lymphomas. After an allogeneic transplant (use of stem cells from someone else), the recipient is given medications to suppress the immune system to reduce the chances the graft will be rejected.

An allogeneic transplant does have some benefits: there are no diseased cells in the donor's blood, and his or her cells may have an anti-cancer effect. Approximately 7,000 allogeneic transplants are performed every year in the United States. The disadvantages of an allogeneic transplant are that it can take time to find a suitable donor; with the exception of some cancer centers, it is offered only to those younger than age 55 (because high doses of chemotherapy with potentially serious side effects are needed); and there is a higher risk of infections and graft-versus-host disease (GVHD, in which the foreign cells [graft] attack the body of the host). GVHD is discussed in more detail beginning on page 169. It is one of the most common reactions to transplants and can affect the intestines, liver, and skin.

The option of transplanting a person's own cells (an autologous transplant) is available in specific situations.

Every year, about 11,000 auto-transplants are performed in the United States. This procedure has several benefits: there is no risk of GVHD; there is no need to wait for a donor; and there is a lower chance of infections. However, autologous transplants cannot be done if the stem cells in the patient's blood or marrow are diseased or if there are not enough cells to transplant. In addition, this type of graft will not have an anti-cancer effect, which can result in a lower chance of a cure in some cases. In general, autologous transplants are performed when patients receive very high doses of chemotherapy and need to have their blood cells replenished.

DID YOU KNOW?

Stem cells are immature, or "blank," cells that are able to become any type of healthy blood cell. In cancer care, transplanted stem cells are used to replace diseased cells in the bone marrow (the tissue inside the bones that forms blood) and prevent cancer from reappearing.

Introduction to Blood Cells

So what exactly are stem cells? Found in all living things, stem cells are a small group of immature (or "blank") cells that develop into all of the blood cells in your body.

Most stem cells are found in the bone marrow, but some, called peripheral blood stem cells, are found in the bloodstream. In up to 80 percent of adults with leukemia, lymphoma, myelodysplastic syndrome, or multiple myeloma, doctors recommend peripheral blood stem cell transplants (PBSCTs). Most autologous transplants are performed with peripheral blood stem cells also. Bone marrow transplants (BMTs) make up about 15 percent of transplants in adults, and umbilical cord blood transplants (UCBTs), in which blood is taken from a newborn's cord, constitute about 5 percent.

Stem cells develop into three main types of blood cells; each type has a different job to do:

- **Red blood cells,** which make up about 40 percent of the blood, carry oxygen to the cells all around the body.
- **White blood cells,** which leave the blood and enter the tissues, are part of the body's immune system; they help to fight infections and other diseases.
- **Platelets,** which are small fragments of cells, halt the bleeding when skin or organs are

injured. They do so by sticking together and forming blood clots.

Treating Cancers With Transplants

Each year, more than 15,000 children and adults in the United States develop some type of condition that can be treated with a stem cell transplant (see box below). Before a transplant is performed, people receive pretreatment with chemotherapy and/or radiation to rid the body of diseased cells and make room for the new healthy cells. The most commonly used chemotherapies are anti-thymocyte globulin, busulfan, cytarabine, fludarabine, melphalan, and thiotepa. They are given in doses that are three to eight times higher than usual. Although the blood and bone marrow are essentially wiped out by these medications, the newly transplanted stem cells will restore the marrow, blood, and immune system.

During the transplant, stem cells are given through a catheter, or tube, placed in the chest or neck by a doctor. Whether the patient or someone else is the donor, that person receives injections of growth factors a few days before the cells are removed, or harvested. These injections help jump-start the production of white blood cells, reduce the chances of infection, and increase the number of cells that can be harvested.

Conditions Treated With Stem Cell Transplants

- Acute myeloid leukemia (most common for allo-transplants)
- Multiple myeloma (most common for auto-transplants)
- Acute lymphoblastic leukemia
- Chronic myeloid leukemia
- Hodgkin lymphoma
- Non-Hodgkin lymphoma
- Myelodysplastic syndromes
- Aplastic anemia
- Other cancers (especially in children)

The cells may be obtained from the donor's blood through a needle in the arm, a catheter or port (in a procedure called apheresis), or from the hip bone in a procedure called bone marrow aspiration. Withdrawing cells from the hip is performed under local anesthesia.

Once the healthy stem cells are introduced into the recipient patient's bloodstream, they travel to the bone marrow, where they begin to produce new white blood cells, red blood cells, and platelets. The growth of these new cells is a process known as engraftment, and it usually takes two to four weeks after transplantation. The goal is for the healthy transplanted cells to recognize the patient's remaining cancer cells, destroy them, and establish themselves in the body to start growing.

After a transplant, many people have to stay in the hospital for four to six weeks so that doctors can keep a close eye on any complications that may emerge. If the transplant is autologous, or if high doses of chemotherapy are not given, hospital stays will be shorter. With the immune system knocked out from the conditioning (or ablation), low levels of white blood cells can lead to infections. Low levels of red blood cells can result in anemia, which makes one tired, pale, and weak. And low levels of platelets lead to bleeding, bruising, or purple spots on the skin, especially on the forearms.

Other possible side effects of transplants include:

- Diarrhea
- Mouth sores
- Difficulty eating
- Problems with the kidneys, liver, lungs, and heart
- Graft failure, in which the stem cells do not survive and mature in the recipient's body
- Rejection of the new cells received from another person.

Transplants and GVHD

The most important skin side effect for those who have had a transplant is called GVHD. It's a condition with a very

> **DID YOU KNOW?**
> Normally, the immune system is supposed to protect the body against foreign invaders, so it sees the transplanted cells as "foreign" and destroys them. To avoid this, doctors suppress the immune system with medicines to avoid graft rejection.

descriptive name: the graft (donated cells) opposes the host and causes a disease. When the donor's T cells (a type of white blood cell that is part of the immune system) face the host's cells, these T cells see them as foreign, so they do what they are born to do: attack unknown cells.

At any time after a transplant, there is a risk of developing GVHD. When GVHD happens within three months of transplantation, it is called acute GVHD. On average, acute GVHD usually occurs around 25 days after transplant. When it happens more than three months or even years later, it is called chronic GVHD. With both acute and chronic GVHD, the skin is the most frequently affected organ.

Doctors take a number of steps to try to prevent GVHD. Transplant doctors try to choose graft donors with a genetic makeup similar to the patient and give medicines to suppress the immune system during the first few months or even years after the transplant. Doctors may also remove the donor's T cells to prevent GVHD (called a T-cell–depleted graft). Although this approach reduces GVHD risk significantly, it increases the

Donors and Graft-Versus-Host Disease (GVHD)

When the Donor Is...	The Percentage of Recipients With GVHD Is...
Sibling (matched)	25 to 40 percent
Identical twin	0 percent
Unrelated (matched)	50 to 60 percent
Umbilical cord	10 to 20 percent
Related or unrelated (partially matched)	70 percent
Any donor (but with T cells removed)	10 percent
Same person (autologous)	0 percent*

These percentages may vary depending on various factors, including the degree of genetic match, a person's age, the type of chemotherapy before the transplant, whether the transplant is free of T cells (so-called T-cell depleted), and whether medications to prevent GVHD were used. Transplant doctors are the best source of information and can determine the risk in individual cases.
*There is controversy over whether GVHD can occur in this setting.

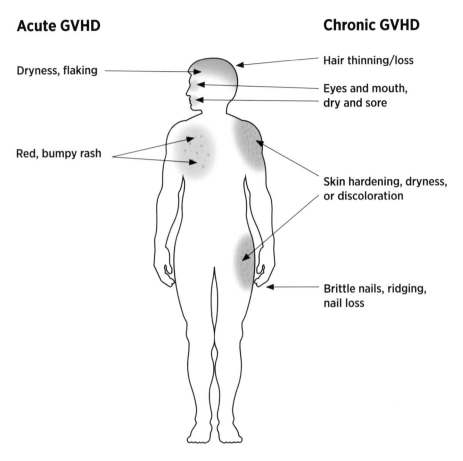

Acute GVHD

Chronic GVHD

Dryness, flaking

Hair thinning/loss

Eyes and mouth, dry and sore

Red, bumpy rash

Skin hardening, dryness, or discoloration

Brittle nails, ridging, nail loss

THE APPEARANCE OF GRAFT-VERSUS-HOST DISEASE
A number of skin, hair, and nail changes are found in both acute and chronic graft-versus-host-disease.

patient's risk of infection, so antibiotics (trimethoprim-sulfamethoxazole), antivirals (acyclovir or valacyclovir), and antifungals (voriconazole or posaconazole) are given during the first few months after the transplant. These medications, as well as the chemotherapy used during the conditioning, can all cause side effects, such as itchy rashes, mouth sores, skin darkening, and sensitivity to the sun. For this reason, it may be difficult for doctors to determine whether a rash after a transplant is GVHD or a reaction to a medication, since they may look similar. Performing a skin biopsy, selectively stopping

DID YOU KNOW?

Approximately 70 percent of transplants for people with cancer are autologous; 30 percent are allogeneic. Most of the time, stem cells are obtained from donors' blood, less frequently from their bone marrow or from umbilical cords.

Q **I'm worried about acute GVHD. What are the risk factors for acute GVHD?**

A Your transplant doctor is the best person to evaluate your chances of developing acute GVHD. Here are some risk factors for GVHD:
- Donor or recipient of advanced age
- A female donor and a male recipient, especially if the woman was pregnant or received a transfusion before
- Donor and recipient are a genetic mismatch
- The patient has advanced cancer at the time of transplantation
- Transplant is unmodified (it contains T cells)
- When certain anti-GVHD medicines cannot be used
- Donor and recipient have different blood types
- Donor cells come from the blood (as opposed to the bone marrow or umbilical cords)

DID YOU KNOW?

In many people who develop a rash after a transplant, a cause (either a medication or GVHD) cannot be found. The treatment, however, is usually the same and in most cases will resolve the rash.

some medications, or using oral or topical immunosuppressive medications may be necessary in these cases.

Approximately one third to one half of people who receive transplants from another person develop acute GVHD; most cases are mild. The risk is slightly higher for those who receive the transplant from an unrelated or mismatched donor. The first signs of acute GVHD are usually a rash, with itching, burning, redness, and small bumps on the trunk and sometimes on the palms or soles. Dry, itchy skin can also appear on the upper body, face, and scalp, which may look like dandruff. This may spread to the trunk and perhaps even the entire body, rarely including the mouth, eyes, and genitals. The skin can blister, but that is extremely unusual. According to a recent study of people with acute GVHD, about 80 percent experienced skin changes. It's also common for people with GVHD to experience diarrhea and liver problems, which are diagnosed through a colonoscopy and blood tests. It is important to remember that transplant doctors have many tools to treat these problems effectively.

GVHD is not the only reason that rashes develop after a transplant. Since people are usually started on many new medicines to fight off infection and to prevent GVHD

Acute GVHD: What It Looks Like

- Dry, flaky skin, especially on the scalp or face but can extend to any other body area
- Redness, rash (bumps and red spots), and itching
- Blistering, especially in the mouth and the genitals
- Sensitivity to the sun, in the form of easy sunburns
- Mouth sores
- Hair thinning or loss

itself, they may experience a rash caused by a medication or even a viral infection. This commonly happens with the use of antibiotics, antifungals, chemotherapies used in the conditioning regimen (cytarabine, fludarabine), or those used to prevent mouth sores (palifermin) and GVHD (anti-thymocyte globulin). Therefore, it's important to tell your doctor if a rash appears, as it could be managed by changing some of the medications or treated with topical or oral corticosteroids and oral antihistamines (the latter in case there is itching). Your doctor may order blood tests, perform a skin biopsy, or stop certain medications to determine the cause of the rash. Even people who receive autologous transplants may develop rashes as a result of medications they are receiving or because their own cells react against their skin, which has likely changed after chemotherapy or radiation therapy.

DID YOU KNOW?

Anti-thymocyte globulins are proteins derived from rabbits or horses. Given before an allogeneic transplant to prevent GVHD, they may cause intense hives and itching.

Grading and Treating Acute GVHD

With treatment, acute GVHD generally lasts for a short time. To determine the type of anti-GVHD treatment, doctors assign grades to acute GVHD.

Grade 1 *Rash consists of red spots and bumps covering less than 25 percent of the skin surface.* Usually treated with topical corticosteroids (fluocinonide, clobetasol) and oral antihistamines (diphenhydramine [Benadryl] or hydroxyzine), if there is itching. Most people usually see an improvement in their condition with these treatments.

Skin Changes After Transplants: It's Not Always GVHD

Not every dermatologic condition experienced after a transplant is GVHD. Skin changes may also be caused by other treatments used as part of the transplant.

Treatment	Side Effect
Radiation	Mouth sores, hair loss, dry skin, skin discoloration
Cyclophosphamide	Acne-like rash, hair loss, mouth sores, skin and nail darkening
Etoposide	Rash, mouth sores
Melphalan	Allergic rash, nail darkening, mouth sores, hair loss
Fludarabine	Itching, rash, mouth sores, hair loss
Cytarabine	Swelling and/or blisters in the hands and feet, sores, dry mouth
Busulfan	Skin darkening, mouth sores, hives, hair loss
Trimethoprim-sulfamethoxazole	Red, itchy rash
Voriconazole	Rash, sensitivity to the sun
Thiotepa	Red rash, itching, skin darkening, hair loss
Anti-thymocyte globulin	Rash, hives, itching, skin swelling on the arms or legs, mouth sores
Tacrolimus or sirolimus	Acne-like rash, skin swelling on the face, mouth sores
Cyclosporine	Skin lumps, acne-like rash, increased hair on the face and body
Prednisone/methylprednisolone	Acne-like rash, stretch marks, easy bruising, accumulation of fat under the skin, increased hair on the face and body
Mycophenolate mofetil	Rash, skin swelling on the arm and legs
Palifermin	Thick, white spots in the mouth, bumpy, itchy rash on the armpits and groin

Mouth sores occur in nearly everyone receiving a transplant. In some cases, eating is affected, and nutrients must be supplied through the veins or a port. One way to reduce mucositis is by using a medicine that stimulates the growth of mouth skin cells (palifermin). Reactivation of oral herpes (cold sores), which is also common, is prevented with antiviral medications.

Grade 2 *Rash consists of red spots and bumps covering from 25 to 50 percent of the skin surface.* Treatment usually consists of oral corticosteroids (prednisone, dexamethasone) for one to two weeks and sometimes even longer, with or without additional medicines to suppress the immune system. About half of the people treated this way will improve.

Grade 3 *Rash consists of red spots and bumps covering more than 50 percent of the skin surface.* Treatment usually consists of oral corticosteroids for one to two weeks and sometimes even longer, as well as other medicines to suppress the immune system. Most people will improve with this treatment.

Grade 4 *Redness covers all of the skin with blisters.* Treatment usually consists of a combination of oral medicines to suppress the immune system and corticosteroids (dexamethasone, prednisone) for weeks to months. At this grade of severity, people are usually admitted to the hospital to receive intravenous medications and control frequently occurring skin infections.

Note When severe GVHD does not improve with the use of oral corticosteroids after two weeks, other medications to suppress the immune system may be added, including alefacept, denileukin diftitox, etanercept, intravenous immunoglobulin, mycophenolate mofetil, pentostatin, sirolimus, and tacrolimus.

Understanding and Treating Chronic GVHD

Chronic GVHD usually occurs around four months after transplantation but may not develop for a year or more, especially if people are on medications that suppress the immune system. The condition generally lasts for a longer time than acute GVHD and is one of the most common problems several years after a transplant. It appears in 15 to 50 percent of people receiving allogeneic transplants. In 70 percent of chronic GVHD cases, the skin is affected, and the skin involvement will determine the overall severity of the condition. About half the time, it follows an episode of acute GVHD that has not resolved. In chronic GVHD, the skin can change in many ways. People can experience skin dryness, color changes, or hardening. Although there is a good chance that a person who has had acute GVHD may go on to have chronic GVHD, the chronic form can appear in those who have never had acute GVHD.

Transplant doctors do many things to try to prevent chronic GVHD, and many options are available to treat it, if it were to appear. If chronic GVHD is severe, the skin may blister and peel, as can happen with a severe sunburn. The skin color may darken, and the texture of the skin may become hard or rough. Sometimes, the skin can become tight and less elastic, especially in areas that have received radiation or are subject to friction, such as under the belt or bra. In some people, hair loss and thin, brittle nails occur. Not only can the skin become dry as

Chronic GVHD: What It Looks Like

- Very dry, thin, or fragile skin
- Tiny, red bumps on the arms and legs
- Purple or red and scaly, round spots or blisters
- Darkening or lightening of the skin
- Redness on the entire skin, including the palms and soles
- Hardening or tightness of the skin in areas, sometimes with swelling, ulcers, or blisters; can look like dimples or cellulite and may limit the movement of joints
- Mouth dryness; whitish or red spots; and sores of the lips, gums, inside the cheeks, and even the tongue
- Nails are affected in 50 percent of people, and changes include brittleness, ridging, thickening, separation, and growth of the cuticles over the nail
- Eye dryness, sometimes with pain; may affect vision
- Dryness in the vagina, which can become narrow; skin can become hard and thin and easily bleed or hurt
- Hair thinning or loss
- Purple spots on the penis; skin can become tight, blocking the flow of urine

a result of chronic GVHD, but also the eyes, mouth, and genitals may show signs of dryness.

To treat chronic GVHD, doctors use medicines that suppress the immune system. But these medications need to be carefully controlled, since they can increase the risk of infections, kidney or bone problems, and reappearance of the cancer. If these drugs don't work, doctors will use other medications (such as imatinib, mycophenolate mofetil, pentostatin, or rituximab) or a procedure called extracorporeal photopheresis (or ECP), in which blood is taken from the body and treated with a chemical and a special light. This treatment removes cells believed to cause GVHD. Another option is phototherapy (or UV light treatment), in which a special light is shone on a person's skin for a few minutes several times a week at a dermatologist's office. Although these rays are similar to those that come from the sun—which doctors normally advise patients to avoid—the treatment is done under controlled circumstances using a special machine under a doctor's supervision.

Grading and Treating Chronic GVHD

As with acute GVHD, doctors grade the chronic form of the condition to determine the best treatment.

Grade 1 *Skin changes (rash, discoloration, redness, bumpy, itching, but no hardening) affect less than 18*

DID YOU KNOW?
About 60 percent of people who develop chronic GVHD will have changes in the mouth (dryness, white or red spots, sores) and eyes (dryness); about 15 percent experience side effects in the genitals (spots, tightness, or dryness).

Q I had a transplant a year ago, and the donor was my sister. Recently, my doctor reduced my immunosuppressive medications, and I noticed red bumps on my skin on top of dark discoloration and dryness. Is this chronic or acute GVHD?

A Although acute GVHD occurs within 100 days of the transplant, red bumps or rash can be found in chronic GVHD, resulting in what doctors call an "overlap" type of GVHD since it has features of both acute and chronic types. Overlap GVHD makes up about 40 percent of cases. Your doctor has many tools to treat "overlap" GVHD.

Useful Treatments for Skin Effects of GVHD

Effects of GVHD	Treatment
Acute GVHD rash	Topical or oral immunosuppressives*
Chronic GVHD (rash)	Topical or oral immunosuppressives*, photopheresis, UV light therapy, imatinib, radiation, acitretin/isotretinoin, rituximab, alemtuzumab, etanercept
Itching	Topical corticosteroids (clobetasol, fluocinonide)
	Oral antihistamines (cetirizine, diphenhydramine, doxepin, fexofenadine, hydroxyzine, loratadine)
	Topical anesthetics (lidocaine, menthol, pramoxine)
	Nerve modulators (aprepitant, gabapentin, pregabalin)
Dryness, flaking	Exfoliant moisturizers (ammonium lactate [AmLactin], lactic acid [Lac-Hydrin], urea, salicyclic acid)
Chapped lips	Topical hydrocortisone or tacrolimus ointment and antibiotic (Polysporin)
Sensitivity to the sun	Sunscreens (broad spectrum with an SPF of at least 15), water-resistant
Darkening skin	Bleaching creams (hydroquinone, azelaic acid, retinoids)
Chronic GVHD (tight skin)	Immmunosuppressive medicines*
	UV light therapy, extracorporeal photopheresis
	Physical therapy
Skin sores	Topical antibiotics (Polysporin)
	Oral antibiotics
	Wound care (by doctor or nurse) and use of dressings (Allevyn, Adhesive, 3M Tegaderm Hydrocolloid)

*Corticosteroids (dexamethasone, prednisone) and other immunosuppressants (cyclosporine, methotrexate, mofetil, mycophenolate, pentostatin, sirolimus, tacrolimus) may be given by mouth; some may be applied directly to the skin.

percent of the skin surface. At this grade, topical corticosteroids or immunosuppressives (tacrolimus) may be effective. For dry, dark areas, exfoliant moisturizers may be useful.

Grade 2 *Skin changes (rash, discoloration, redness, bumpy, itching, or skin hardening) affect 19 percent to 50*

Useful Treatments for Nail Effects of GVHD

Effects of GVHD	Treatment
Brittle nails	Biotin (Appearex 2.5 mg or 2,500 mcg a day)
	Orthosilicic acid 10 mg a day (BioSil)
	Nail strengtheners daily (CITRA Formaldehyde-Free #3, OPI Nail Envy Natural Nail Strengthener, China Glaze Nail Strengthener & Growth Formula, Sally Hansen Hard As Nails)
Ridges	NailTek Foundation daily
Discoloration	Dark nail polish such as OPI Lincoln Park after Dark or Black Cherry Chutney, China Glaze Evening Seduction, Sally Hansen Pat on the Black, Polished Mama Date Night
Loss	Consider silk wraps at a salon

percent of the skin surface. The skin can still be pinched, even if it has hardened. At this grade, oral medicines to suppress the immune system are usually required.

Grade 3 *Skin changes (rash, discoloration, redness, bumpy, itching, or skin hardening) cover more than 50 percent of the skin surface; thick skin that is unable to be pinched; sores, severe itch, or tightening of the joints.* At this grade, oral immunosuppressives are required, possibly with antibiotics and in some cases other methods such as phototherapy or extracorporeal photopheresis.

Chronic GVHD of the mouth is graded separately as mild (symptoms do not affect eating); moderate (symptoms somewhat limit the ability to eat); severe (symptoms severely limit the ability to eat).

Chronic GVHD of the eyes is graded as mild (dry eyes that require drops less than three times a day); moderate (dry eyes that require drops more than three times a day or special plugs); severe (dry eyes with pain, affecting work or the ability to see). It is important to make an appointment with an ophthalmologist if any eye discomfort develops.

Useful Treatments for Mouth Effects of GVHD

Effects of GVHD	Treatment
Sensitivity	Rinse with an alcohol-free mouthwash (Biotene)
	Avoid hot, cold, or spicy foods; citrus fruits; mint; and sodas
	Use toothpaste for sensitive or dry mouth (Biotene, Sensodyne)
Sores	Topical triamcinolone, tacrolimus ointment, viscous lidocaine four times a day
Painful white or red areas	Mouthwashes medicated with dexamethasone and nystatin. Swish around the inside of the mouth for four minutes and then spit out. Repeat four to six times a day. Clotrimazole lozenges (troches) four times a day or miconazole buccal tablets daily for yeast infections
Dryness	For dry mouth, artificial saliva sprays (Mouth Kote, Biotene), gels or liquids (Biotene Oral Balance, Numoisyn) or lozenges (Numoisyn, up to 14 a day). For severe cases, cevimeline (30-mg tablets three times a day), pilocarpine (5-mg tablets three times a day)
	Fluoride protection to prevent cavities when the mouth is dry (Colgate PreviDent 5000 Plus, wash or gel)

Useful Treatments for Hair Effects of GVHD

Effects of GVHD	Treatment
Hair loss/thinning	Minoxidil (Rogaine 5%)/finasteride (for men only)
	Biotin (Appearex 2.5 mg or 2,500 mcg a day), orthosilicic acid 10 mg a day (BioSil)
	Wigs, extensions, or hair thickeners (diCesare Thicken Hair Builder, DermMatch Topical Shading, or Toppik Hair Building Fibers) or sprays and powders that cover the scalp (Top Coverage for Bald Spot and Thinning Hair, Bumble and Bumble Hair Powder)
Scalp redness or itching	Topical corticosteroids (betamethasone or clobetasol foam, fluocinonide solution)

Useful Treatments for Eye Effects of GVHD

Effects of GVHD	Treatment
Dryness	Dry eyes can be alleviated with artificial tears used up to four times a day (Systane Ultra High Performance Lubricant Eye Drops, GenTeal Severe Dry Eye Relief Lubricant Eye Gel, Visine Tears Lubricant Eye Drops)
	Ophthalmologist may insert a plug in the corner of the eyelid to retain tears
Dryness or pain	Corticosteroid or immunosuppressive drops prescribed by an ophthalmologist

The Skin After a Transplant: Handle With Care

If you have had a stem cell transplant and notice any changes in your skin, hair, nails, or mouth, be sure to tell your transplant doctor right away. Your doctor can determine whether these changes are a result of a medication or GVHD. The tables "Useful Treatments for GVHD" on pages 178–181 list the different types of medications that may be prescribed to prevent complications.

DID YOU KNOW?

People who develop GVHD are at a lower risk for the original cancer to reappear.

If you have chronic GVHD, it's important to:

- Have regular skin examinations to monitor any growing or changing spots. The risk of skin cancer is higher in people with GVHD, so skin checks every year are mandatory.
- Care for any ports or catheters to prevent infections.
- Test any sores or ulcers for infection.
- See your dentist regularly so he or she can examine your mouth for any changes. Any new spots or growth in the mouth that persists or appears after the transplant must be evaluated by an oral surgeon.
- Have a vaginal exam (for women). GVHD can create dryness and narrowing, but other conditions may be the cause as well, such as estrogen deficiency or infections.

Safety Tips After Transplants

Use these tips, especially during the first six months of treatment:

- Wash your hands with soap and water or a liquid sanitizer after using the bathroom, cooking, changing diapers, going to public places, or handling animals or plants.
- Bathe or shower daily with a gentle, fragrance-free soap (Aveeno, Basis, Cetaphil, Dove, Vanicream)
- Do not wear contact lenses during the transplant period. Ask your doctor when you may wear your contact lenses again.
- Do not rupture any skin blisters
- If a family member has a rash from receiving a vaccine, avoid contact with him or her and inform your transplant doctor.
- Latex condoms should be used, especially in people who are not monogamous.
- Before handling catheters or ports, wash your hands. Protect the port or catheter with an adhesive dressing or barrier, cleaning with chlorhexidine.
- Inspect your skin and report any rash, pain, redness, swelling, or other skin changes to your transplant team.
- Use electric clippers to remove hair, instead of shaving.
- Use fragrance-free detergents when washing your clothes.
- Avoid public hot tubs, ponds, lakes, or rivers.
- Protect yourself against the sun, and apply a broad-spectrum water-resistant sunscreen with an SPF of at least 15.

DID YOU KNOW?

Hand washing or use of hand sanitizers should be frequent, especially during the first six months after the transplant. Use a moisturizer on the hands after washing or using a sanitizer.

For more details on skin side effects, see Chapters 3 ("Taking Care of Dry Skin") and 4 ("How to Stop the Itching"); for more on nail side effects, see Chapter 5 ("Keeping Nails Healthy"); for information on sun protection, see Chapter 10 ("Sun Safety"); and for more on hair loss, see Chapter 6 "(Handling Hair Changes").

Researchers and transplant doctors are continuing to search for better ways to prevent and manage GVHD. Many doctors and nurses work together to ensure safety and the best possible results.

Nutrition is also key to taking care of your skin during and after a transplant. Eating well improves the quality of the skin, your immune system, and your overall health. Ask your doctor to recommend a registered dietitian who can help advise you. And remember to stay active if possible, and seek help from a physical medicine and rehabilitation doctor or physical therapist if there are any limitations on your ability to perform daily activities, work, or exercise.

THINGS TO REMEMBER

- Stem cells are a small group of immature (or "blank") cells that develop into all of the different blood cells in the body. Transplantation is a procedure that gives healthy stem cells to a person whose cells are not working properly.

- Approximately 300 registered patients search the worldwide registry network for unrelated bone marrow donors every month. Almost one million people in the United States are living with, or are in remission from, leukemia, lymphoma, myelodysplastic syndrome, or multiple myeloma. Tens of thousands undergo stem cell transplants every year throughout the world.

- Certain types of cancer, including leukemias, lymphomas, and multiple myeloma, can be treated with transplants.

- Chemotherapy and/or radiation therapy are used with transplants to destroy any cancer cells in the bone marrow or blood and to decrease the chance that the person receiving these new cells will not react against them.

- The side effects of pre-treatment chemotherapy and radiation therapy are similar to those for standard cancers, except they may be more severe.

- Graft-versus-host disease (GVHD) is a frequent complication of transplants, in which the transplanted cells react against the patient's healthy cells. GVHD affects primarily the skin, lungs, liver, and intestines.

- Eighty percent of people who have acute GVHD and 70 percent of those with chronic GVHD will experience changes in their skin.

- Skin changes in acute and chronic GVHD include rash, redness, itching, discoloration, tightness, and dryness. Hair can thin or fall out, the mouth can become dry or sore, eyes can become dry, and the nails can become brittle.

- Medications and lifestyle changes can ease the discomfort of skin changes caused by the transplant. After transplants, care must be taken to maintain healthful habits for the skin.

CHAPTER 10

Sun Safety

Your oncologist has probably advised you to avoid the sun and to use sunscreen whenever you spend time outdoors. But if you have ever walked through the sunscreen aisle at a pharmacy, you know how overwhelming it can be. There are many products with a variety of terms to describe them: SPF, UV-A, UV-B, broad-spectrum, sunblock, sunscreen, water-resistant, sweat-resistant, etc. Which is the best sunscreen for you? And how can you avoid the sun and still go outdoors?

The information in this chapter will help you choose the right products and sun-safe behaviors. You'll learn more about:

- Protecting your skin from the sun's rays during and after cancer treatments
- Sunscreen use and key ingredients
- Sun-protective clothing
- Cancer treatments and medications that can increase your risk of sunburns or skin cancer

Sun Basics

Despite what you may have heard or read, tanning is not good for anyone, especially for people living or having lived with cancer. Overexposure to the sun—whether it's often or just once in a while—can lead to sunburns, aging of the skin, spots, and skin cancer. Any part of your body, including your ears, scalp, hands, and lips, can burn. The sun can also damage your eyes, which are ex-

DID YOU KNOW?

Most anti-cancer medications as well as some antibiotics, antifungals, and non-steroidal anti-inflammatories make you more likely to get a sunburn.

The Skin Type Classification System: How Sensitive Is Your Skin?

Type I: Always burns, never tans, high skin cancer risk
Found in people with white pale skin, blue/green eyes, blonde/red hair

Type II: Burns easily, tans just a little, high skin cancer risk
Found in those with fair skin, blue eyes, dark blonde hair

Type III: Burns first, then tans, low skin cancer risk
Occurs in people with dark white skin, light brown/green eyes, light brown hair

Type IV: Burns very little, tans easily, very low skin cancer risk
Affects those with olive/light brown skin, brown eyes, and brown hair

Type V: Almost never burns, tans dark, extremely low skin cancer risk
In those with brown skin, brown eyes, brown/black hair

Type VI: Never burns, tans always, almost no skin cancer risk
Found in people with dark brown/black skin and eyes, black hair

DID YOU KNOW?

The US Environmental Protection Agency estimates that the sun causes 65 percent of melanomas and 90 percent of other types of skin cancer.

tremely sensitive to its ultraviolet light. That is why it's important to wear sunglasses that are made specifically to protect against the sun's harmful ultraviolet (UV) rays. Ultraviolet rays (also known as UV radiation) are a form of energy from the sun. Other forms of energy from the sun are visible light and heat. Whereas light allows us to see and heat prevents us from being cold, UV radiation is not only invisible but much stronger: it damages living organisms, including the cells in our skin, by altering their DNA (genetic material).

Signs and symptoms of sunburn usually appear within a few hours after sun exposure. However, it may take a day or more to know the full extent and severity of a sunburn. Skin type is one of the many factors that determine the degree to which a person gets sunburned and the risk of skin cancer. Dermatologists divide skin types into six categories, ranging from Type I (always burns) to Type VI (never burns). (See the table above.) Other factors include length of time exposed to the sun and geographic location. People closer to the equator and those at higher altitudes receive the highest amounts of the sun's rays. People with dark skin are less likely, but not completely protected from, developing skin cancers, premature skin aging, and sunburns. The sun can damage their skin, causing white or dark spots or other skin discolorations.

Most people are unaware of the amount of sun exposure they receive. You don't have to be lying on a beach or by the pool to be exposed to the sun: daily activities such as shopping, going to work, and running errands all result in sun exposure. In addition, everyone is exposed to low levels of UV rays from fluorescent lamps used for indoor lighting and UV lamps used in insect traps. You should also note that certain oral or topical medications and even contact with plants such as figs, dill, parsley, carrots, lime, and celery might make it more likely that you will burn in the sun. See the table on page 188 for some common examples. Increased sensitivity to the sun from medications can occur in anyone, no matter how light or dark the skin is.

> **DID YOU KNOW?**
>
> Cosmetics combined with sunscreen (SPF) will not affect the protective value of sunscreen contained in them. They have the great advantage that most people apply them every day.

How Much Sun Is Too Much?

The following items can alert you to the level of UV ray exposure

Name	Description
Sol ALERT personal UV detectors (MDSolarSciences)	Wristband or UV card that changes color in response to UV rays
www.mdsolarsciences.com (877) 301-5355	Packaged with every MDSolarSciences sunscreen; can only be obtained this way
Personal UV (Advanced Safety Devices)	Handheld, battery-operated device that displays the UV index and recommends the proper sunblock or tanning lotion by SPF type
www.safety-devices.com (866) 216-8700	Pricey but accurate
UV Index (National Weather Service and the United States Environmental Protection Agency)	Web-based information showing the strength of solar UV rays on a scale from 1 (low) to 11+ (extremely high)
www.epa.gov/sunwise/uvindex.html	Free; also available in apps for mobile phones

Medications/Products Associated With an Increased Risk of Sunburn

Antibiotics	Ciprofloxacin, doxycycline, levofloxacin, minocycline, moxifloxacin, nalidixic acid, tetracycline, trimethoprim-sulfamethoxazole
Antifungals	Griseofulvin, voriconazole
Anti-malarial medications	Chloroquine, hydroxychloroquine
Anti-pain and anti-inflammation medications	Celecoxib, diclofenac, ibuprofen, nabumetone, naproxen, piroxicam
Diabetes medications	Chlorpropamide, glipizide, glyburide, tolazamide, tolbutamide
Gastric medications	Ranitidine
Heart/blood pressure medications	Amiodarone, furosemide, hydrochlorothiazide
Dermatologic medications	Acitretin, isotretinoin
Psychiatric medicines	Alprazolam, amitriptyline, chlordiazepoxide, chlorpromazine, desipramine, imipramine, thioridazine
Vegetables and plants (if they come in contact with skin)	Carrots, celery, figs, lime, parsley, parsnips
Blood-stimulating drugs	Epoetin alfa
Vitamins/herbs	St. John's wort, pyridoxine (vitamin B$_6$)
Anti-cancer medications	All-*trans*-retinoic acid (ATRA), bexarotene, capecitabine, cetuximab, dacarbazine, dasatinib, erlotinib, fluorouracil, gefitinib, imatinib, leuprolide, methotrexate, nilotinib, paclitaxel, panitumumab, vandetanib, vemurafenib
Topical ingredients	Tar (in some medicated creams or roofing materials)

Q I take an anti-cancer medication daily in pill form and it makes me sensitive to the sun. I went out for a walk and now I have a really painful, itchy sunburn, with some blisters. What should I do?

A With certain medications, sunburns can develop even after a few minutes of sun exposure, even if you are in the shade. If this happens, it's important not to stop your treatment but to inform your doctor or dermatologist. In the meantime, take a cool shower or bath, then apply a topical corticosteroid (ideally a prescription strength, otherwise use an over-the-counter hydrocortisone cream). Take an anti-inflammatory such as ibuprofen (Advil) and an anti-itch medicine such as diphenhydramine (Benadryl), unless your doctor advises against using them. Drink plenty of fluids, and don't break or pick any blisters or scratch your skin.

How Do Sunscreens Work?

Sunscreens absorb, reflect, or scatter the sun's UV rays, which are divided into three types, based on the amount of energy they have and the damage they can cause to living beings: ultraviolet A (UV-A), ultraviolet B (UV-B), and ultraviolet C (UV-C). Fortunately, the most harmful UV-C rays do not reach the earth's surface, since they are blocked by the ozone layer in the atmosphere. Only UV-A and UV-B rays reach the earth. UV-A rays cause aging of the skin, sunburns, and skin cancer. UV-B causes tanning and is also largely responsible for skin cancer. Sunscreens provide either physical or chemical protection from UV light.

Physical sunscreens form a physical barrier to UV rays, an opaque film that blocks the rays before they can reach the skin. These sunscreens contain minerals such as zinc oxide or titanium dioxide, which protect against both UV-A and UV-B rays. The original formulations of physical sunscreens were white and gritty when applied. The newer formulations use tiny mineral particles (called nanoparticles) and blend more with the skin tone. They are also less noticeable and smoother. Between 30 and 70 percent of sunscreens use nanoparticles, which are considered safe by regu-

DID YOU KNOW?

Some topical ingredients can cause a skin allergy to the sun, such as PABA (found in some sunscreens), fragrances (musk, sandalwood oil), chlorhexidine and hexachlorophene (found in some skin cleansers), triclosan (used in some toothpastes), ketoprofen (a pain reliever), and the anti-viral acyclovir (for cold sores).

I am getting chemotherapy for lung cancer, but I want to be able to go on vacation to a warm, sunny place and walk outside. Do I have to stay inside all the time?

No. If you want to be outside or go somewhere tropical, you can definitely do that. However, it is important to be rigorous about following sun-protective measures. Use a broad-spectrum sunscreen with an SPF greater than 15; reapply it every two hours; wear protective clothing and a hat and sunglasses; and avoid direct exposure to the sun without protection between 10 am and 4 pm.

DID YOU KNOW?

A greater risk of sunburn occurs in places close to the equator and when the sun is directly overhead; in areas with sand, snow, or water, which reflect the rays; and in locations at a higher altitude, where the atmosphere is thinner.

latory agencies. The best way to find a physical sunscreen is to look for "zinc oxide" or "titanium dioxide" in the list of ingredients. Not only are they safe to use, they have shown antibacterial effects on the skin.

Chemical sunscreens use various compounds to absorb UV rays before they can cause any damage. These compounds convert the UV energy into heat (which may be why some sunscreens make your skin feel warm). They contain one or more ingredients such as avobenzone or oxybenzone, which absorb UV-A or UV-B rays. For greater protection, chemical sunscreens often contain more than one ingredient to protect against both types of rays. A combination of avobenzone and oxybenzone can be found in Helioplex (in Neutrogena products) or Active Photobarrier Complex (in Aveeno products). This combination protects against UV-A and UV-B rays. Ecamsule (Mexoryl SX, found in Anthelios sunscreen) is a newer sunscreen, which protects against both UV-A and UV-B rays.

Despite what many people believe, allergies to sunscreens are rare. The most common ingredients causing allergies are oxybenzone, benzophenone, and para-aminobenzoic acid (PABA). If you suspect you are allergic to a sunscreen, apply a small amount behind your ear or on your forearm and keep it covered with a small adhesive dressing for two days. When you remove the dressing, if there is any redness, itching, or swelling, this indicates that you are allergic and should avoid using this sunscreen. You can then use a different type of sunscreen or have an allergy patch test done by a dermatologist. Patch testing involves the application of various substances to the skin on the back, under an adhesive tape that is left in place for 48 hours. Then the skin is examined for redness or rash, and the dermatologist will advise how you can avoid the allergy-causing products.

Many factors can make sunscreens less effective. They include high humidity, sweating, drying or rubbing your skin with a towel, and exposure to water when swimming or showering, for example.

Sunscreen Safety

Laboratory studies have shown that sunscreens remain on the surface of the skin and are not absorbed into the body. So at the amounts normally used, sunscreens are not harmful to your health. No link has been found between the use of sunscreens and breast cancer, for instance. Sunscreens undergo rigorous safety tests before they can be approved by the U. S. Food and Drug Administration so they can be sold to the public.

Because the sun converts substances in our skin into vitamin D, using sunscreen may cause a vitamin D deficit. This vitamin plays many important roles in the body: it helps ensure bone health and may reduce the risk of getting certain types of cancer. To make sure you get enough vitamin D, you can supplement your diet with a daily dose of 1,000 IU (international units) of vitamin D. If you do use supplements, doctors recommend you take no more than 2,000 IU per day. People at high risk for insufficient amounts of vitamin D are the elderly, those with dark skin, those who are overweight, and those who stay indoors or live in colder climates with little sun exposure. If you are concerned about your level of vitamin D, ask you doctor to perform a simple blood test. Supplements or increased

DID YOU KNOW?

A simple way to tell how much of the sun's rays you are getting is to look at your shadow: if your shadow is taller than you (in the morning and late afternoon), your UV ray exposure is probably low, but if the shadow is shorter, (around noon), you may be getting too much UV, so seek shade and protect yourself.

Q How much and how often do I need to apply sunscreen?

A Sunscreen should be applied at least 30 minutes before going outside and every two hours thereafter (or every 40 to 80 minutes if swimming or sweating, or as indicated on the label). To cover all exposed parts of the body, a recommended application is about one ounce (35 milliliters)—the amount in a shot glass or the size of a golf ball. Remember the teaspoon rule: use more than half a teaspoon on each of these areas: your head and neck, left arm, and right arm. Use more than one teaspoon on each of these areas: your chest and stomach, right leg, and left leg. Gently massage into the skin until the product disappears, leaving the skin smooth.

DID YOU KNOW?

Sunscreen sticks are good to use on lips and around the eyes. Up to 90 percent of lip cancers occur on the lower lip. That's because more of the sun's rays reach that area. Also, using the sunscreen stick on your eyebrows helps prevent sunscreen from dripping into your eyes when you sweat.

intake of certain foods that contain vitamin D may be recommended (see table below).

The important thing to bear in mind is that people living with cancer should make it a priority to avoid complications and hence care for their skin, and that includes protection against harmful radiation from the sun. It's certainly best to avoid sunscreens with ingredients that may irritate your skin such as fragrances, dyes, or preservatives, especially if they are known to cause an allergic reaction.

Eat or Drink Your Vitamin D

Food	IU
Cod liver oil, 1 tablespoon	1,360
Sockeye salmon, cooked, 3 ounces	447
Tuna fish, canned in water, drained, 3 ounces	154
Orange juice fortified with vitamin D	137
Milk, vitamin D–fortified, 1 cup	120
Liver, beef, cooked, 3.5 ounces	49
Egg, 1 large (vitamin D is in yolk)	41
Swiss cheese, 1 ounce	6

Most people like the way in which chemical sunscreens spread easily and blend on the skin. But it's understandable if you feel you do not want to add more chemicals to your body. So you can choose physical sunscreens, which contain tiny metallic particles of zinc or titanium that block the sun's rays. These types of products may give you more peace of mind. Vanicream sunscreen (www.psico.com) contains zinc oxide and is specifically designed for sensitive skin, since it is free of any fragrances or perfumes. Sunscreens containing the minerals zinc and titanium are also available in many brands.

Shedding Light on Protection Terms

Sun Protection Factor (SPF) indicates how long you can stay in the sun without burning from UV rays. For example, if you have skin that burns in 20 minutes, when you use a sunscreen with an SPF of 15, you would multiply 20×15, which equals 300 minutes, or 5 hours. Theoretically, this is the amount of time you could stay in the sun without burning if you use an SPF 15 sunscreen. This rating system does not account for the amount of sunscreen that hasn't soaked into the skin or the amount that is rubbed off by clothing, sweating, or swimming.

Ultraviolet Protection Factor (UPF) is the international standard for rating UV protection added to clothing. It measures how well clothing protects you from sunburns. UPF takes into account the type of fabric used, its weave, weight, and color as well as how much of the skin the fabric covers. A UPF of 40 or higher has an "excellent" rating, the highest possible. A fabric with this rating blocks more than 98 percent of UV rays.

The UV Index, developed by the U. S. National Weather Service and the U. S. Environmental Protection Agency, indicates the strength of solar UV rays on a scale from 1 (low) to 11+ (extremely high; see page 194). It predicts these levels based on factors such as ozone, latitude, elevation, time of year, and time of day. You can use the UV Index as a guide for when it's best to avoid sun exposure. The UV Index can be found at

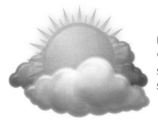

UV Index less than 2 is considered low. Protection with a three-inch brim hat, sunglasses, and sunscreen, on exposed areas, is advised. You can safely stay outside.

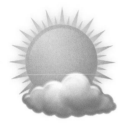

UV Index 3 to 5 is considered moderate and requires some protection. Seek shade during midday hours. Wear sunscreen and a hat with a three-inch brim and sunglasses.

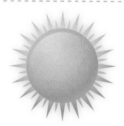

UV Index above 6 is considered high and requires extra protection. Seek shade during midday hours. Wear sunscreen and protective clothing, including a shirt, a hat with a three-inch brim, and sunglasses. Use a broad-spectrum sunscreen that protects against both UV-A and UV-B rays.

DID YOU KNOW?

Because it may take up to 24 hours for a sunburn to fully develop, you can't always count on the look or feel of your skin during a day outside to tell you when you have had too much sun.

www.epa.gov/sunwise/uvindex.html. There, you can also sign up for e-mail or smartphone updates.

Hypoallergenic sunscreen is one that causes fewer allergic reactions. These sunscreens are made for people with sensitive skin or allergies (Vanicream [www.psico.com], MDSolarSciences [www.mdsolarsciences.com], and Blue Lizard Australian Sunscreen Sensitive).

If you like to be tan, fake it using self-tanners. These products give your skin a bronze glow through the ingredient dihydroxyacetone (also known as DHA), derived from sugar. It is safe, and there are many options to choose from. The method of application is key, in order to achieve a smooth natural look. For more information on self-tanners, see Chapter 11, "Using Cosmetics to Look and Feel Better." A word of caution: with the ex-

Sun-Protective Clothing: We've Got You Covered

Brand	Hats	Clothes	M/W/C	Where to Get It	Comments
Bloqwear		✓	M/W	www.bloquv.com (866) 611-bloq (2567)	UPF 50, mostly active wear, limited variety
Coolibar	✓	✓	M/W/C	www.coolibar.com (800) 926-6509	UPF 50+, excellent designs and styling, most comprehensive variety of clothing, full-body coverage
EcoStinger		✓	M/W/C	www.ecostinger.com (888) 291-5008	UPF 50+, only swimwear but excellent variety that covers the body
MDSolarSciences	✓	✓	M/W/C	www.mdsolarsciences.com (877) 301-5355	UPF 50+, limited variety, shorts available, UV Index detector
Sunday Afternoons	✓	✓	M/W/C	www.sundayafternoons.com (888) 874-2642	UPF 50+, good variety and prices, available for all members of the family, limited availability of pants
Sun Precautions	✓	✓	M/W/C	www.sunprecautions.com (800) 882-7860	UPF "excellent," great variety of products and styles, long-lasting fabrics
Sun Protection Zone	✓	✓	M/W/C	www.sunprotectionzone.com (714) 894-0646, Ext. 206	UPF 50+, modern designs for all members of the family, UVSunSense UV Exposure Monitoring Wristband in stock, no pants
Tilley	✓	✓	M/W	www.tilley.com (800) 363-8737	UPF varies between different fabrics, great variety of products and styles
UNIQLO	✓	✓	W	www.uniqlo.com customerservice@uniqlo-usa.com	UPF 50+, stylish designs for women
Wallaroo Hat Company	✓		M/W/C	www.wallaroohats.com (888) 925-2766	UPF 50+, great variety of hats for the entire family

M/W/C = men/women/children

ception of a few products (Clarins Self Tanning Milk SPF 6, Clarins Delectable Self Tanning Mousse SPF 15, and Peter Thomas Roth Bronze Instant Mineral SPF 30), self-tanners (unlike a tan) will not protect you against the sun's UV rays. So you must still use sunscreen.

Light spectrum   The sun's rays consist of a continuous range of waves that reach the earth's surface. For human health, we are concerned with UV-A and UV-B.

How to Choose and Apply the Right Sunscreen

Not all sunscreens are the same. Here are some general guidelines for choosing the best one for you:

Select a broad-spectrum sunscreen with an SPF of at least 15. Broad-spectrum products provide protection against both UV-A and UV-B rays. Check the ingredient labels for zinc, titanium, ecamsule, or a combination of avobenzone plus oxybenzone (Helioplex or Active Photobarrier Complex).

Look for sunscreens labeled "water resistant," which offer some protection against exposure to water, during swimming or sweating. Sunscreens can no longer be labeled "waterproof" because all sunscreens wash off to some extent.

Terms that can no longer be used on sunscreen product labels include "sunblock" (no product actually blocks all UV rays), "immediate protection," and "all-day" (no sunscreen lasts all day). However, some sunscreens, such as Neutrogena Wet Skin Sunblock Spray SPF 30, can be applied on skin that has become wet from swimming or sweating.

Avoid tanning oils and lotions. Many do not contain sunscreen. Such products are required by law to clearly state on the label whether they have an SPF factor. Take time to read the fine print on product labels.

Understand the different uses for different forms of sunscreen. Sunscreens are available as creams, gels, lotions, sprays, and wax sticks. Lotions and creams are the most commonly used types of sunscreens and are best for individuals with dry skin,

Your Sunscreen Should...

- Have a sun protection factor (SPF) of at least 15

- Provide broad-spectrum protection against both UV-A and UV-B rays

- Contain one of the following ingredients: the mineral zinc oxide or titanium dioxide, Ecamsule (Mexoryl SX), or avobenzone plus oxybenzone (Helioplex or Active Photobarrier Complex)

- Not be chosen based on other additives that are touted as beneficial to the skin, such as vitamin A, vitamin E, or botanicals, for example. Also, it is important to avoid PABA, as many people can be allergic to it.

- Be labeled "water resistant," especially if you will be swimming or sweating

- Include a section on "Drug Facts" listing all the ingredients

but gels are preferred by people with oily skin or with acne. Gels also tend to wash off more easily with water. Although a sunscreen spray is easy to apply, usually not enough of it is used. The only instances where a spray is recommended is for hairy areas (the scalp and male chest). Hair sunscreens are not ideal but may be useful for people who have lots of hair or for those who are going swimming or are sweating and can't wear a hat. Hair sunscreen can usually be applied on wet or dry hair and will not come off with simple immersion in water.

Apply sunscreen liberally 30 minutes before going outdoors, even on cloudy days. It takes 20 to 30 minutes for sunscreen to be absorbed by the skin, so don't wait to put it on until you're already outside.

Reapply sunscreen every two hours or sooner as needed. If you are sweating or swimming, the sunscreen will wash off, so you need to apply it every 40 to 80 minutes. Note that when you dry your skin with a towel, it removes more than 80 percent of the sunscreen on your skin.

> **DID YOU KNOW?**
>
> Only half as many people who should use sunscreen actually do so. And of those who use sunscreen, most people apply half or less of the recommended amount.

My cancer is colorectal, not skin cancer. Do I really need to worry about sun exposure when I have other things to worry about?

The real reason for protecting yourself against the sun is that chemotherapy and other medicines can make you more sensitive to the sun, causing severe, painful sunburns. Also the sun suppresses your skin's immune system, making it more susceptible to skin infections. For example, cetuximab and fluorouracil, both medications used against colorectal cancer, can increase your sensitivity to the sun.

Protect all exposed parts of the body. Clothing, including hats, is also a good way to protect against the sun. Clothing limits the amount of skin exposed to the sun. You can purchase clothing that provides sun protection with specially treated fabric that contains a UPF. The most popular brands are Tilley, Coolibar, and Solumbra (from Sun Precautions); they have many different types of designs. If you want to give your own clothes a UPF, you can add sunscreen with the special laundry detergent SunGuard (www.sunguardsunprotection.com). The active ingredient in SunGuard is Tinosorb, a physical sunscreen that blocks more than 96 percent of the sun's harmful rays. A typical white cotton T-shirt provides a UPF of 5, but SunGuard increases the UPF to 30. When added to your

How Well Do Fabrics Protect Against the Sun's Rays?

Property	Excellent Protection	Poor Protection
Construction	Tightly woven	Loosely woven
Fabric weight	Heavy	Light
Fiber type	Wool, polyester	Cotton, polyamide silk, polyacrylic
Color	Dark, bold	Light, pastels
Moisture	Dry	Wet
Fit	Loose fitting	Tight fitting

UPF Shielding by Clothing: The Ultraviolet Protection Factor (UPF)

UV Protection	UV Rays Blocked	UPF Number
Good	93 to 96 percent	15, 20
Very good	96 to 97 percent	25, 30, 35
Excellent	More than 98 percent	40, 45, 50, and above 50

UPF = Ultraviolet Protection Factor; UV = ultraviolet

clothes during a laundry cycle, SunGuard offers protection that lasts for up to 20 washes.

Choose moisturizers and/or cosmetic products with an SPF of at least 15. The US Food and Drug Administration advises people living with cancer to moisturize with sunscreen-containing products because anti-cancer medicines may make patients more sensitive to harmful UV rays. It's best to avoid any potentially irritating chemicals such as fragrances or dyes. Women have a number of choices in cosmetics that contain sunscreen. Some products for men also combine a moisturizer and a sunscreen.

If you are using a moisturizer as well as a sunscreen, the moisturizer should go on first, then the sunscreen, and finally the makeup. If you are also using a topical medication prescribed by your doctor, it should be applied before everything else.

DID YOU KNOW?

Water-resistant sunscreens will protect after two immersions in water of 20 minutes each. Very water-resistant ones will stay on after 4 immersions of 20 minutes each.

Sun Protection Factor (SPF): The Degree of Sunscreen Protection

An SPF of	Will Block This Percent of UV Rays
4	70 percent
8	88 percent
15	94 percent
30	97 percent
50	98 percent

Secrets to Applying Self-Tanning Products

- Before applying the tanning products, use a moisturizer, especially on the knees and elbows
- Make sure your skin is not wet or sweaty before you apply
- Avoid the palms, soles, armpits, and groin
- Apply lightly on the elbows and knees
- Apply it evenly, to avoid streaks
- Start with a small area, so you can see how dark you will get

The following are among the preferred self-tanners:
- Jergens Natural Glow Express Body Moisturizer (www.jergens.com)
- Au Courant Sunless Tanning Mousse and Lotion (www.aucourant.com)
- Decléor Aroma Sun Expert Self-Tanning Milk (www.decleor.com)
- Clarins Self-Tanning products (www.clarins.com)
- Origins The Great Pretender shimmery self-tanner for body (www.origins.com)
- St. Tropez Self Tan Bronzing Mousse (www.sttropeztan.com)

DID YOU KNOW?

The risk of skin cancer is higher in people who have received stem cell transplants, medications that suppress the immune system, and radiation.

Avoid insect repellent and sunscreen combinations. There are more than 20 products that combine insect repellents and sunscreen. Of note, the most commonly used insect repellent is DEET, and its safety has been demonstrated over the past 50 years: less than 25 cases of side effects have been reported. In fact, the American Academy of Pediatrics recommends the use of DEET in children older than 2 months. There is minimal absorption of DEET into the body, but when repellents are mixed with sunscreen, their absorption into the body may be increased, and consequently their side effects may be greater. Also, the sun-protective ability of sunscreens is decreased by about one third when they are mixed with insect repellents. Since sunscreens need to be applied generously every two hours, and repellents applied sparingly and no more frequently than every six hours, using combination products is not feasible and impractical. Therefore, it is not recommended to use combination sunscreen and insect repellent products. In this case, the recommendation is for using sun-protective clothing and applying an insect repellent or applying sunscreen and using a repellent that you don't need to spray on, such as OFF! Clip-On Mosquito Repellent.

The Other Side of the Sun: Self-Tanners

For people who like to look tanned, the only safe alternative to sun exposure or tanning beds is to use self-tanners. A note of caution: There are no pills that are approved to stimulate, enhance, or develop a tan; taking such pills could be dangerous to your health.

Self-tanning products have come a long way since the days when they made people look orange and had a funny smell. Now, self-tanners give a beautiful bronze glow and in some cases even help conceal blemishes or imperfections on the skin. The ingredient that allows for this color is dihydroxyacetone (also known as DHA), a by-product of sugar with no known negative or toxic effects on human health when applied to the skin. The DHA adheres to dried-up cells on the skin surface, resulting in a chemical reaction that gives the brown color.

Practice makes perfect, especially when applying self-tanners, so start with small areas and allow the product to dry before putting on your clothes (usually at least 15 to 30 minutes). In that way, you can avoid staining your clothes or getting streaks on your skin. Keep in mind that no matter how much self-tanner you apply, it will not protect you against the sun's rays as a sunscreen would.

The Facts on Sun Protection

Despite all the recommendations and the care that must be taken, it is important for people to enjoy their hobbies, their life, and the ability to spend time with their families, even in sunny places. The idea then is not to avoid any activities or locations, but to use sensible measures. Keep in mind that when sunscreens are ineffective, it is because people don't use enough of them or don't reapply them as often as they should. Also, sun-protective hats and clothing are not used properly or frequently enough. When you use sunscreens and sun-protective clothing, you can enjoy your life outdoors to the fullest.

THINGS TO REMEMBER

- When receiving chemotherapy, targeted therapies, or radiation, it's very important to apply a broad-spectrum sunscreen generously, with an SPF of at least 15, every two hours. Also, use protective clothing and avoid being outside unprotected. Be sure to wear sunglasses with lenses that protect your eyes from UV rays.

- Physical (mineral) sunscreens are more opaque, whereas chemical sunscreens are more greasy.

- Some people can be allergic to ingredients in sunscreens, most commonly PABA and oxybenzone.

- For people who don't like to apply sunscreen, there are options such as sun-protective clothing and hats. You can also wash your own clothing with SunGuard detergent, which makes clothes resistant to UV rays.

- The American Academy of Dermatology recommends using vitamin D supplements, rather than engaging in sun exposure, if your vitamin D levels are low.

- Self-tanners do not provide protection against UV rays. And although tanning from the sun does protect against sunburns, it is not recommended as a method of protection from additional sun exposure.

- You may feel safe indoors without protection, but window glass (as found in homes or cars) lets UV-A rays go through, so sunburns and other negative effects of UV rays can still happen, even when inside a home or car.

- Certain medications may make it more likely that you will get sunburned, so check with your doctor about the medications you are receiving.

- Although sunscreens and clothing do not provide total protection, it's important to enjoy your life outside, as there are emotional and physical benefits of activities during the daylight, especially if they take place with loved ones.

CHAPTER 11

Using Cosmetics to Look and Feel Better

osmetics are products used to improve the appearance or scent of the body. They include creams, powders, foundations, blushes, lotions, powders, lipstick, mascara, nail polish, and hair dyes. Many people living with cancer may benefit from the enhancing or concealing effects of cosmetics. But many are also concerned about the chemicals in cosmetics and the negative effects they may have. This chapter explains which cosmetics are safe and effective in improving skin changes that result during or after cancer treatments. Information on nail and hair cosmetics has been included in Chapter 5 ("Keeping Nails Healthy") and Chapter 6 ("Handling Hair Changes").

Except for the colors in cosmetics and hair dyes, the U.S. Food and Drug Administration (FDA) does not certify or approve what goes into cosmetics before they are sold to the public. The FDA strongly urges cosmetic manufacturers to conduct safety tests on their products, but voluntary testing is done by only about 40 percent of companies. Cosmetic companies also have the option of voluntarily reporting injuries caused by their products. It's also important to note that, as long as they don't promise a permanent change in the skin, hair, or nails, makers of cosmetics do not have to prove that their products reduce wrinkles, improve skin tone, or any of their other countless claims, many of which are baseless. In most cases,

DID YOU KNOW?

The U.S. Food and Drug Administration (FDA) defines cosmetics as products intended to be applied to the human body for cleansing, beautifying, promoting attractiveness, or altering the appearance, without affecting the body's structure or function.

it's up to the person who uses these products to judge their worth and effect.

Fortunately, many products are safe to use during and after cancer treatments. Many people—both men and women—find that using cosmetics to improve their appearance makes them feel better. A person's appearance plays a role in his or her sense of self and the perceptions of others. Although we all know that what matter most are personality, morals, and family, every little bit of help to make life more social, active, happy, and full makes a big difference during challenging times. This chapter will help give you the tools to put your best face forward!

Looking Good and Feeling Better

In 1987, a woman receiving cancer treatment was so distressed by the changes in her physical appearance, she would not go outside of her hospital room. Her doctor asked the president of the Personal Care Products Council if he could organize a makeover for the woman. Calls were made and a makeup artist came to the hospital with cosmetics, transforming "not only the woman's look, but also her outlook. She felt happier, less burdened, and laughed for the first time in weeks."

That first effort blossomed into a national program called **Look Good...Feel Better**. It's available in every

I'm worried that my foundation or blush will clog my pores and cause acne. Is it safe to use makeup during chemotherapy, or will it make any rash or acne get worse?

I encourage people to use concealing cosmetics, including foundation or powders, to cover acne, rashes, or blemishes caused by anti-cancer medicines. Acne or rashes caused by these medicines will not be affected by cosmetics. However, when you use a new product or suspect a cosmetic is causing a reaction on your skin, apply the makeup on a small area behind the ear and leave it on overnight, to make sure it doesn't trigger acne or rash.

state, the District of Columbia, and Puerto Rico (see www.lookgoodfeelbetter.org). The success of the program illustrates how important a role cosmetics can play in improving self-image, especially for people living with cancer. When you look good and feel good, despite what you may be going through, you take control of your life again. That's an important part of the healing process.

Although Look Good...Feel Better is a program for women, men too can benefit from the lift in their spirits that cosmetics can provide—there are products like "guyliner" and "manscara." In 2010, *The New York Times* reported on the boom in sales of men's skin care products, most notably, those made by a company called Mënaji, the official skin-care line for the Prostate Cancer Foundation. Mënaji bills itself as a masculine and undetectable line of cosmetics and skin care products. The products don't add color to men's eyelids or cheeks but they do mask imperfections such as dark circles under the eyes or blotchy skin.

For most people, any type of cosmetic can be used at any point during treatment. In this chapter, you'll learn more about choosing and using the best products and which ingredients to avoid. But always talk with your doctor about whether using cosmetics during treatment is medically safe for you, and that will depend on the type of treatment you are receiving and

DID YOU KNOW?

Women in ancient Egypt used cosmetics to accentuate their eyes; 400 years ago, Europeans used beauty patches to hide smallpox scars on the face.

I use a good facial cleanser, but I still get occasional acne-like breakouts from my cancer treatment. Should I use a scrub or something else to clean my face better?

Acne-like breakouts caused by certain types of chemotherapy, targeted therapy, or corticosteroids are not caused by dirt or insufficient face cleansing. Using a gentle cleanser containing 2 percent salicylic acid or 5 percent benzoyl peroxide may help reduce inflammation and decrease any bacteria on your skin. Avoid using loofahs, scrubs, or exfoliating brushes, as they can lead to inflammation and possibly infections. If needed, use a clean washcloth.

any pre-existing skin conditions such as itching, infections, and dryness.

If your doctor tells you that the chemotherapy or targeted therapy you are receiving does not lead to skin side effects, there is no reason why you can't continue using cosmetics during treatment. However, it is important to tell your doctor or nurse if an area where you have been applying a cosmetic shows any of the signs of an allergy (redness, swelling, or itching) or infection (redness, swelling, discharge, or pain).

What Is a Cosmetic?

The Food, Drug, and Cosmetic Act defines cosmetics by their use: "Articles intended to be rubbed, poured, sprinkled, or sprayed on, introduced into, or otherwise applied to the human body...for cleansing, beautifying, promoting attractiveness, or altering the appearance." Among the products included in this definition are skin moisturizers, perfumes, lipsticks, nail polishes, eye and facial cosmetics, shampoos, permanent waves, hair dyes, toothpastes, and deodorants.

Some products that have two intended uses are considered to be both cosmetics and drugs. For example, a

Q After receiving chemotherapy, I got an itchy red rash on my eyelids, which a dermatologist called an allergy to eyeshadow. I've been using this product for many years. Is it possible that I can be allergic to something I've used for a long time?

A I am convinced that chemotherapy or stem cell transplants can cause new allergies to develop. These allergies can occur during or after chemotherapy or a transplant. In the case of stem cell transplants, it is possible that if a donor had an allergy, it was "transmitted" to the recipient. In any event, the first step is to avoid the suspected product and to treat the allergic rash with a topical corticosteroid. The second step is to identify the culprit, either through a "use test," which you can do yourself, or a "patch test," which is performed by a dermatologist or allergist. (See the box on the next page.)

Skin Allergy Testing: The Patch Test

Performing a patch test is a good way to identify and prove a possible allergy to a substance. The first step is to bring to your dermatologist's office any cosmetics, fragrances, eye drops, creams or lotions, nail polish, or anything else you may be applying to your skin. Special sticky tapes that have potential allergy-causing ingredients will be applied to your back for two days, after which the doctor will remove them and examine the skin on your back for a reaction. When you have the tapes on, you should not get your back wet by exercising or showering (use a washcloth instead). A positive test reaction will look like a small red rash, which is sometimes itchy. Three visits to the doctor's office are needed for this test, and you should not take oral corticosteroids within two weeks before the test. At the final visit, your doctor will tell you what things you may or may not be allergic to, and what products to avoid.

shampoo is a cosmetic because it is intended to cleanse the hair. But if it's an anti-dandruff shampoo, it is also a drug because it treats a flaky scalp. It may be important to remember this difference while you are being treated for cancer, because a cosmetic product that contains a "drug" has the potential to interact with anti-cancer medications you are taking (although this is extremely unlikely). The FDA does not have a pre-market approval system for cosmetic products or ingredients, with the important exception of color additives. On the other hand, drugs are subject to FDA approval and must be tested to show they are both safe and effective.

DID YOU KNOW?

The symptoms of skin allergies to cosmetics are usually redness, dryness, and itching.

Choosing and Using Cosmetics

If you decide to use cosmetics to hide side effects such as skin discoloration, pimples, dark circles under the eyes, or loss of eyebrows and eyelashes, the best advice is to try one product at a time. Use it for several days before adding another product, just to make sure each new cosmetic doesn't cause a rash or other skin reaction. You can also do a "use" test; apply just a small amount on the inside of your forearm or on a quarter-sized area behind your ear (most places that sell cosmetic products will let you sample them) and cover it with a bandage. Leave it on for two days, and if you see any redness, blistering, or itching, you are allergic to it and should not use it. It's a good idea to follow up with a skin allergy specialist (a dermatologist) to determine which of the many ingredients in the cosmetic is causing the problem. (Note: makeup removers can also be the source of an allergy.) Even if a product is labeled "hypoallergenic," "unscented," "for sensitive skin," "all-natural," "organic," or "non-comedogenic," it can still cause an allergy or acne. These labels simply indicate that ingredients known to cause allergies have been removed, and so they are less likely to cause a reaction. These labels are medically unproven and are simply part of the marketing strategy. However, generally, well-known companies conduct safety testing of their products.

A dermatologist can perform a "patch" allergy test on your skin for a definitive answer. The eyelids are the most common areas where people develop allergies to cosmetics, so the ingredients of all products used have to be looked at carefully. Some of the ingredients that cause allergies are meant to prevent even another complication: skin infections resulting from germs growing in the cosmetics. Signs of a skin infection include redness, swelling, pain, and discharge of fluid. Although cosmetics rarely cause infections, a person receiving chemotherapy may have both a weakened immune system and fragile skin. So it's important to change the cosmetics regularly, as a precaution.

To Prevent Infections: Change Your...

Mascara	Every three months
Powder blush	Every two years
Cream blush	Every year and a half
Eye shadow	Every year
Lipstick and lip gloss	Every two years
Lip and eye pencils	Every two years (sharpen at every use)

Whether or not you use cosmetics, it's important to continue moisturizing your skin (see Chapter 3, "Taking Care of Dry Skin"). That's because some cosmetics can dry the skin, and dry skin often leads to a wrinkled appearance or blemishes. Using moisturizers won't get rid of wrinkles, but they will improve the overall appearance and texture of your skin.

If you are applying several products on your skin, it's best to follow the sequence shown below:

DID YOU KNOW?

Only about 10 percent of the 10,500 ingredients used in cosmetics have been tested for safety. The FDA does not routinely test cosmetics for their safety, and companies are allowed to use any raw material they like, barring a few prohibited chemicals.

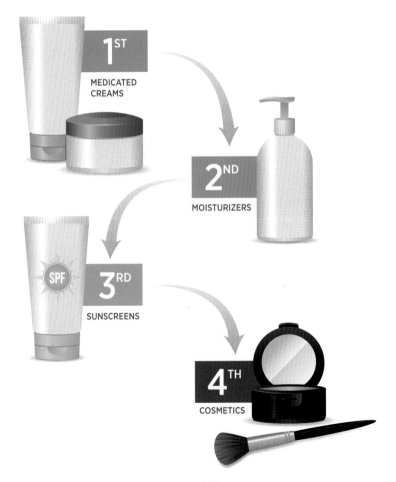

1ST MEDICATED CREAMS

2ND MOISTURIZERS

3RD SUNSCREENS

4TH COSMETICS

RECOMMENDED SEQUENCE FOR APPLYING PRODUCTS TO YOUR SKIN
Because moisturizers create a barrier, you want to use any medications first, so they have the best chance of being absorbed into your skin. And because makeup can smudge, it's best to apply it last.

Read the Label

Some commonly used cosmetics contain ingredients that can cause unwanted reactions. The tables below and at right list the ingredients that can cause allergic reactions, irritation, and infections.

Applying Cosmetics the Right Way

A Few General Points...

The key words for cosmetic application are light and healthy. Although your tendency might be to overcompensate and apply heavy makeup, it will result in an unnatural look. Apply cosmetics with a light touch. To project a radiant, healthy look, accentuate the positive and conceal the negative.

Be sure to clean your face regularly. Don't pull, tug, or scrub your face too hard. Aggressive cleansing with scrubs or loofahs can strip away the remaining natural oils, so use a washcloth instead. The friction caused by scrubbing or rubbing your skin can cause inflammation, resulting in loss of skin tightness. It's best to use lukewarm water and soap-free, water-soluble face cleansers, which gently wash away cosmetics and oil without drying out the skin.

For the Face

As discussed in Chapter 3, moisturizing your skin is extremely important, especially the skin on your face.

Types of Cosmetics to Avoid
"All natural," "organic," or unpreserved products (they may contain infectious germs)
Those made with botanicals such as arnica, camphor, eucalyptus, ginseng, menthol, tea tree, and wintergreen
Products that use abrasives to "exfoliate," including loofahs, salt scrubs, and sugar scrubs, since friction on the skin causes inflammation
Talcum powder used in the genital area, since it has been associated with ovarian cancer

Types of Ingredients to Avoid

Acetone
Alcohols (including ethanol,
  isopropyl alcohol, SD alcohol)*
Benzidine-based dyes
2-Bromo-2-nitropropane-1,3-diol
  (BPND)
Butylated hydroxyanisole
Butylated hydroxytoluene
4-Chloro-ortho-toluidine
Cinnamon
Clove
Coal tar (found in inexpensive
  mascaras)
Colophony
Dibutyl phthalate
1,4-Dioxane
Di-tert-butylhydroquinone
Formaldehyde or formaldehyde
  releasers such as DMDM hydantoin

Grapefruit
Imidazolidinyl urea
Lanolin derived from sheep's wool
Lavender
Metals (especially nickel, bismuth
  oxychloride, mica)
4,4'-Methylenebis
Mint
n-Nitrosodiethanolamine (NDELA)
Parabens**
Peppermint
Phenylmercuric acetate
Potassium sorbate
Quaternium-15
Sodium lauryl sulfate (levels higher
  than two percent)
Wintergreen
Witch hazel

*Cetyl alcohol, steryl alcohol are not irritating.

**There is some controversy as to whether these products are dangerous.

Modified, with permission, from Draelos (2001).

Make it part of your daily routine. The best time to apply a moisturizer is right after washing. Pat the skin dry and apply moisturizer while the skin is still damp. When using a moisturizer along with your cosmetic, apply a color-correcting moisturizer before using any makeup on the face. Recommended products are Eucerin Redness Relief Daily Perfecting Lotion SPF 15 or Clinique Even Better Skin Tone Correcting Moisturizer SPF 20 (for daytime), Eucerin Redness Relief Soothing Night Creme or Clinique New Moisture Surge Intense Skin Fortifying Hydrator (for nighttime), and L'Oreal Studio Secrets Professional Secret No.1 Magic Perfecting Base for use under makeup.

The first makeup to apply is a concealer, which should match your skin tone as closely as possible. If it's too light or too dark, it will draw attention to any

When You're in Treatment...Tips on Choosing Cosmetics

Because chemotherapy, targeted therapies, radiation, and stem cell transplants can all affect the normal functioning of the skin and make it more sensitive, you need to carefully select the products you use. Here are some helpful tips:

- Throw out old cosmetics and buy new products.
- If possible, buy cosmetics with no more than 10 ingredients.
- Select cosmetics without allergy-causing sunscreens (such as PABA esters or methoxycinnamate).
- Make sure your makeup can be easily removed with water, since removing waterproof cosmetics can dry and irritate the skin; use them only when necessary (if, for instance, you don't want your mascara to run because you plan on crying at a wedding!).
- When possible, choose powder or cream cosmetics over lotion formulas. Facial foundations should be of the cream/powder variety. If liquid, they should be based on silicone derivatives (cyclomethicone, dimethicone).
- Use an eyebrow powder or gel to thicken eyebrows.
- Avoid eye shadows that are creams, sticks, or pencils. Powder eye shadow is easier to remove with water, which is less irritating to delicate eyelid skin than makeup remover.

Modified from Draelos (2001).

DID YOU KNOW?

If you wear contact lenses, it is better to insert them before you apply eye cosmetics. In that way, you'll avoid smearing the makeup and possibly getting it in your eye when you handle the wet lens.

skin problem rather than hide it. The salespeople in cosmetic sections of department stores or in specialty cosmetic stores can help you find the best color for the most natural look.

When applying concealer, use a method called stippling: place a small dot of concealer on a cosmetic sponge and dab it on your face, blending it around the area of the skin flaw as you go. *Note: if you are allergic to latex, make sure that the sponge is not made from that substance. You can use your fingertips instead of the sponge.* Repeat by applying small dots and stippling until you have covered the imperfection. Concealers are especially useful in hiding blemishes or pimples that result from targeted therapies (see Chapter 2, "All Rashes Are Not Created Equal," for more on these treatments).

The second makeup to apply is the foundation. When purchasing foundation, it's a good idea to sample the shade on your neck instead of your hand. This is the skin that the foundation will need to match, and it may be very different from the skin on your hand. By combining two foundation colors, you can achieve the most natural appearance. Neutral colors (tan or cream) and a matte finish offer the best coverage.

Apply the foundation by dotting and stippling with a damp sponge, beginning in the center and working outward and upward in gentle, circular strokes. Be sure to blend the product over the entire face, including on the eyelids and under the jaw line and chin. Concentrate on the areas under the eyes and around the nose, as dark circles or blemishes tend to appear there.

If you have oily skin, face powders also cover any skin flaws, and they have the added benefit of controlling oil. Powders give a matte finish and make the skin feel smooth. Originally, face powder was applied over a moisturizer to function as a powdered foundation. But liquid foundations have largely replaced powdered foundations, because they adhere better to the skin and last longer. However, for people who wish to have sheer coverage with excellent oil control, a powdered founda-

DID YOU KNOW?

Fragrances are protected by trade secret laws, which allow manufacturers not to list the ingredients contained in colognes or perfumes.

Q **I've been using a brand of face powder that I really like. Should I buy everything else for my skin from that brand?**

A A brand doesn't assure that all of its products are effective or will satisfy your expectations. Furthermore, certain brands have many different lines of cosmetics. Larger brands are usually recommended because they have more resources to conduct safety testing and more people have probably used them successfully. You should note that more expensive cosmetics don't necessarily work better. Everyone's skin is different, so you will have to try different products to determine which ones are best for you.

Makeup Trend: Cosmeceuticals

We all want to age gracefully, but many people would prefer that the effects of aging—wrinkles, dark or white spots, loose skin, gray hair—not show quite so starkly. Enter cosmeceuticals, products that promise to enhance the look of facial skin by reversing or preventing aging. Practically speaking, that's nearly impossible. And because no long-lasting benefits have been proven with the use of cosmeceuticals, you need to adjust your expectations and watch your wallet, as these products can be expensive. Still, some medications that have also been labeled cosmeceuticals do show an effect in some clinical studies, as detailed below.

Cosmeceuticals That Have Shown an Effect in Clinical Studies*

Drug name	Effect
Azelaic acid	Lightens skin, reduces acne
Benzoyl peroxide	Reduces acne
Bimatoprost	Promotes eyelash growth
Eflornithine	Reduces facial hair
Hydroquinone	Lightens skin
Mequinol	Reduces dark spots on back of hands
Minoxidil	Increases hair growth
Sunscreens	Prevents sunburns, skin aging, and cancer
Tretinoin, tazarotene	Reduces wrinkles, lightens skin, removes blackheads

*Some of these cosmeceuticals will be effective only at prescription-strength concentrations, so ask your dermatologist.

tion might be preferred. Look for products that offer full coverage and are translucent—that is, they allow light to pass through. If you decide to use powder instead of a liquid foundation, be sure to apply moisturizer for your skin type, allow it to dry, and then apply the powder.

If you have particularly dry skin, face powders are not generally recommended because they draw attention to any skin flaws. It's better to use just a light dusting of loose powder if you prefer not to use liquid foundation.

When it comes to blush, less is definitely more. Too much blush can make you look flushed and flustered instead of showing a healthy radiance.

For the Lips

During and after cancer treatment, the lips can become dry and cracked. So it's important to maintain the condition of your lips to reverse any side effects and enhance your appearance. To do so, you need to choose effective lip care products.

Moisturize frequently (at least four times a day) with a thick ointment such as petroleum jelly (Vaseline), Vaniply Ointment, or Aquaphor Lip Repair Ointment. If lips are red and burn or itch, it's important to apply a corticosteroid ointment, such as hydrocortisone 1% (Cortizone-10) or 2.5% (Hytone) twice daily.

Many cases of severe lip dryness and irritation can be caused by an allergy, so try using a toothpaste from Tom's of Maine or Arm & Hammer. Avoid lipsticks, lip pencils, chewing gum, flavored dental floss, mouthwash, and licking your lips, as saliva can irritate the skin. If the problem persists, talk with your dermatologist about having a patch test for allergies.

For women, a creamy lipstick can keep the lips moist as well as attractive. But make sure you only apply lipstick when your lips are healed, especially if they are cracked or blistered from treatment. You can use a lip liner and lipstick to define and highlight the beauty of your lips. Choose a lip liner that is the same shade as your lips or your lipstick. Lip liners work well with lipsticks because they can prevent the color from "bleeding" and help protect against sun exposure.

To use lip liner, begin on the upper lip with short strokes to define the outer edge of the lips, keeping your lips closed and relaxed as you go. Next, line the lower lip, working from the center to the corners. Use a lip brush to fill in the lines of your lips with lipstick. For a natural look, blot lips with a tissue.

> **DID YOU KNOW?**
> More than 60 percent of women have sensitive skin, so it is important to be careful when you apply any new cosmetic.

For Eyes Only

Applying a cosmetic to your eyes can be the most satisfying, the most difficult, and the most problematic—all at the same time. Skin allergy experts have determined that up to 12 percent of cosmetic reactions occur on the eyelids. If you tend to have dark circles under your eyes, most people focus eyeliner, eye shadow, and mascara on the upper lid only. This will draw attention away from the lower lid and better highlight your eyes. Also, you can use a matte-style concealer that has a color similar to the rest of your facial skin (Clinique All About Eyes Concealer, Cover FX Camouflage Concealer, Conceal Rx, Physicians Formula Physicians Strength Concealer). In cases where dark circles become a significant cosmetic issue, an evaluation by a dermatologist is advised. He or she can rule out an allergy, use a laser treatment, or perform a small surgical procedure called blepharoplasty.

Begin with eyeliner, which comes in two varieties: liquid and pencil. Liquid eyeliners contain latex and are more likely to cause infections (or rash if you are allergic to latex). Pencils are safer and more popular. It's important to sharpen the eyeliner pencil before each application to reduce the possibility of infection. Depending on the shape of your eyes and the look you want, you can line the top and bottom lids or just the top. Experiment to see what works best for you. Hold

Q Should I apply one of the specially labeled "eye creams" for the area around my eyes?

A Most of the time, the only difference between creams labeled for the eyes and other areas is the packaging, labeling, and the higher price. The most important features of a moisturizing cream for the face (and the area around the eyes) are not irritating, retains moisture, and provides sun protection (for the daytime cream). However, if you have dark circles around the eyes, using a tinted cream to conceal them would be a useful feature of your eye cream.

I've almost completed my chemotherapy, and I would like to get a facial. Is this something I can do, and will it improve the appearance of my skin after chemotherapy?

 Most of the time, facials use products and machines that have unproven effects for any skin condition. However, facials do relieve stress and make people feel pampered and cared for. But it's important to be cautious, as the hygiene of some of these procedures is not up to medical standards, and the masks may have ingredients that cause allergies. Going to a licensed aesthetician is always a must.

your liner as you would a pencil and line your eyelids as close to the lash line as possible. Follow the shape of your eyes, but be careful not to get your liner too close to the inner corners of your eyes. To soften the look, lightly smudge the line with a Q-tip or your finger.

Then apply eye shadow to highlight and brighten your eyes. One common approach is to use three shades: a medium shade near the lash line, a dark shade from the crease of the eye to the brow bone, and a light shade at the brow bone. Neutral colors work best for the daytime, and bolder colors are best for evening. Make sure each color fades gradually and seamlessly into the next.

Mascara is a wonderful way to thicken, darken, and lengthen eyelashes. It has been used for thousands of years. Today, there are several formulations: water-based, solvent-based, and a mixture of both. Water-based mascaras are easy on the eyes and well tolerated, but they may run with sweating or tearing. They also contain a preservative (usually parabens) to prevent bacterial contamination. Although water-based mascara is less likely to cause allergies, people with allergies to parabens should avoid it. Solvent-based (waterproof) mascara doesn't run and is less likely to carry bacteria, but it can irritate the eyes, and removing it requires a special mascara remover. Mascara should not be shared with other people and should be discarded

DID YOU KNOW?

People with contact lenses or frequent eye infections should use waterproof mascaras or disposable mascara wands.

every three months to prevent bacterial growth. Take care to apply mascara mostly on the tips of the lashes to prevent irritation to the eyelid.

If your eyelashes are still growing back, you may want to hold off on using mascara. Consider using the prescription drug bimatoprost, to increase the length and thickness of your eyelashes, which can be done during or after chemotherapy. For thin or lost eyebrows, crayons applied in a feathery motion may do the trick until your eyebrows return to full strength. Brow powders can create natural-looking eyebrows if yours have not fully returned after chemotherapy. Use eyebrow stencils (www.eyebrowz.com) to create the eyebrow shape that looks best on you.

Going Natural and Free

The Personal Care Products Council (PCPC) created the Cosmetic Ingredient Review (CIR) System, by which an expert panel reviews the safety of ingredients in cosmetics and makes the results public. To date, less than 15 percent of ingredients have been reviewed.

According to the FDA, natural ingredients are those that are extracted directly from plants and animals. However, this does not necessarily mean that they are clean, pure, or good for the skin. Most of the botanicals and their effects have never been tested to prove their claims.

On the other hand, fragrance-free cosmetics from large companies such as Almay and Clinique have several advantages: fragrances, which are one of the most common causes of allergies, have been removed, and the cosmetics will have undergone extensive testing on many people to make sure that the risk of allergy or irritation is minimal to none.

Resources
The Campaign for Safe Cosmetics
www.safecosmetics.org
This coalition effort was launched in 2004 to protect the health of consumers and workers by securing the

Natural Choices

Cosmetics

Aubrey Organics (www.aubrey-organics.com)

Bare Escentuals (www.bareescentuals.com)

Burt's Bees (www.burtsbees.com)

Lavera (www.lavera.com)

Perfumes

DSH Perfumes (www.dshperfumes.com)

Essence of Vali (www.essenceofvali.com)

InFiore (www.infiore.net)

Intelligent Nutrients (www.intelligentnutrients.com)

Jurlique (www.jurlique.com)

Tsi-La Organics (www.tsilaorganics.com)

corporate, regulatory, and legislative reforms needed to eliminate dangerous chemicals from cosmetics and personal care products.

Cosmetic Ingredient Review
www.cir-safety.org

This organization thoroughly assesses the safety of ingredients used in cosmetics in an open, unbiased, and expert manner and publishes the results in the peer-reviewed scientific literature.

Cosmeticsinfo.org
www.cosmeticsinfo.org

This website includes scientific information on ingredients most commonly used in cosmetics and personal

DID YOU KNOW?

Foundations and concealers can be used to hide rashes or blemishes caused by cancer treatments. Cover FX has the best variety of corrective cosmetics, and they can even be matched to your skin tone.

Fragrance-Free or Sensitive-Skin Cosmetic Choices

Almay (www.almay.com)

Clinique (www.clinique.com)

care products in the United States. The PCPC and its member companies sponsor this site to provide consumers with comprehensive safety information on cosmetics and personal care products so people can make informed purchases.

Skin Deep
www.ewg.org/skindeep

As part of the Environmental Working Group (a founding member of the Campaign for Safe Cosmetics), Skin Deep helps protect the health of consumers and workers by requiring the health and beauty industry to phase out the use of dangerous chemicals and replace them with safer alternatives.

Women's Voices for the Earth Campaign for Safe Cosmetics
www.womensvoices.org

This national organization works to eliminate toxic chemicals that affect women's health. Its aim is to change consumer behaviors, corporate practices, and governmental policies.

Look Good...Feel Better
www.lookgoodfeelbetter.org

This non-medical, brand-neutral public service program teaches beauty techniques to cancer patients to help them manage the appearance-related side effects of cancer treatment.

Lindi Skin and Evolife
www.lindiskin.com
www.evolife.com

These companies produce skin care products that have been tested with people living with cancer in mind. Their product lines include skin, mouth, nail, and hair moisturizers, washes, and dressings, with the goal of alleviating discomfort from chemotherapy and radiotherapy. Some of their products have been used in clinical studies, showing some benefit in specific conditions induced by chemotherapies.

Additional Reading

These books are an excellent source for cosmetic use and application in people living with cancer:

- *Facing the Mirror With Cancer: A Guide to Using Makeup to Make a Difference* by Lori M. Ovitz
- *Ramy Gafni's Beauty Therapy: The Ultimate Guide to Looking and Feeling Great While Living with Cancer* by Ramy Gafni

A Final Word on Cosmetics

To sum up, the long-standing myth that cosmetics cannot be used during chemotherapy, radiation therapy, or after transplants is not supported by any medical evidence. However, it's best to understand the ingredients in cosmetics and your sensitivity to them and to use common sense. It *is* possible to feel and look as good as you can, both during and after cancer treatments.

Bear in mind that for people living with cancer, the skin becomes very sensitive, so anything that comes in contact with the skin may irritate it, even products that never posed a problem before. It's always a good idea to test products on a small area behind your ear or the underside of your forearm for one day, then watch for any signs of itching or redness, which suggest an allergy or irritation. This same care of your skin applies to the washes or soaps you use to clean yourself with, as well as the detergents you use to wash your clothes (fragrance-free soaps and detergents are best). Clothing is also something that needs to be carefully selected. Opt for soft cotton clothing that doesn't bind.

DID YOU KNOW?

It is possible to develop allergies to cosmetics at any time, even if you have been using them for years. In fact, new allergies appear in many people after they've had chemotherapy.

THINGS TO REMEMBER

- Your health care team can offer you the best advice on whether you can use cosmetics during cancer treatment. Visit a dermatologist if you would like additional information about products or allergies.

- Clean the skin on your face and remove makeup by using a gentle cleanser that can be used with lukewarm water, instead of makeup removers, astringents, or scrubs.

- The major cause of wrinkles are UV rays from the sun, not dry skin.

- No oral vitamins or supplements have been shown to improve skin appearance.

- It's a good idea to test all cosmetics before you use them to find out whether you are sensitive or allergic.

- Natural or organic products are not always better or safer than synthetic products. The key is to use fragrance-free or hypoallergenic products that have been through extensive testing and used by many people.

- You don't need to buy expensive skin care products to achieve a desired effect on your skin. In fact, studies have shown that expensive products are no better than their inexpensive counterparts.

- Cosmetics may hide certain facial side effects associated with cancer treatments, such as rashes, scars, or skin discoloration from anti-cancer medications, radiation, surgeries, or injections.

- Many cosmetic products contain ingredients that people with cancer should avoid; be sure to read the product labels.

- If you are allergic to latex, beware of sponge applicators made from that material. Also, be careful with cosmetics containing avocados, mangos, papayas, kiwis, peaches, and melons, as there may be a cross-reaction.

- To prevent darkening or staining of the white part of the eye, avoid applying eyeliner to the inner lower lid.

- Alcohol is used as an antiseptic in creams or lotions and can dry the skin when used excessively or in susceptible people.

- The terms "unscented," "dermatologist-tested," "all-natural," "organic," or "cosmeceutical" do not guarantee that the products are any more effective or safe.

CHAPTER 12

Especially for Cancer Survivors

Remarkable advances in chemotherapy, targeted therapies, surgery, and radiation therapy have resulted in more people living longer and being cured of their cancer. As a result, more emphasis has been placed on maintaining quality of life, such as by minimizing the effects of treatment on the skin and even on improving one's appearance. In a survey of cancer survivors, skin conditions were considered the most important of the unexpected side effects of treatment. After receiving chemotherapy, most survivors said they were affected by the degree of skin dryness and irritation and nail problems they experienced. Although most of these side effects go away once treatments are finished, some may persist for several months or years.

Because most people are not aware that treatments can cause skin changes, few survivors consulted a dermatologist before they started chemotherapy. Ideally, a dermatologist should be part of your health care team from the beginning of treatment if there are any pre-existing skin conditions or if the cancer treatment is known to cause significant dermatologic effects. But even after treatment, survivors having skin problems can benefit from seeing a dermatologist who can help with any lingering skin, hair, or nail concerns. It is important to tell your oncologist about any treatments that your dermatologist may recommend. Also, your dermatologist will need to know the specifics of when

DID YOU KNOW?

Being a cancer survivor begins at the time of diagnosis and extends for the balance of life. This definition, now the norm, was written by the National Coalition for Cancer Survivorship.

and how your cancer was treated, so it's a good idea to bring your medical records to your appointment. There's no such thing as sharing too much information with your doctor, when it comes to your health.

In this chapter you will learn more about:

- Skin, hair, and nail issues experienced by survivors as a result of anti-cancer medicines, surgery, and radiation therapy
- The best ways to improve or prevent skin cancers and lasting side effects
- Recommended evaluations to be performed by a dermatologist, according to cancer type
- Information specific to childhood cancer survivors

Surviving Persistent Skin Discoloration

In most people, side effects of cancer therapies are temporary. Of the more than 900,000 people receiving more than 70 different anti-cancer medications (including chemotherapy, targeted therapies, and hormonal treatments) every year, very few experience persistent skin side effects that cannot be managed. About

Medications That May Cause Persistent Skin Discoloration (Red, White, or Dark)

Arsenic trioxide	Etoposide	Mercaptopurine
Bleomycin	Estradiol	Methotrexate
Busulfan	Estramustine	Mitoxantrone
Capecitabine	Fluorouracil	Paclitaxel
Carmustine	Gefitinib	Panitumumab
Cetuximab	Ifosfamide	Pazopanib
Cyclophosphamide	Imatinib	Procarbazine
Dactinomycin	Ipilimumab	Sunitinib
Dasatinib	Interferon	Thiotepa
Docetaxel	Lenalidomide	Toremifene
Doxorubicin	Mechlorethamine	Vinblastine
Erlotinib	Medroxyprogesterone	

Survivors: Know Your Risk

- Childhood cancer survivors have a skin cancer risk six times higher than the general population. The risk is higher for those who have received radiation and will increase over years to decades after the initial cancer treatment.
- Skin cancers are more frequent in people who received allogeneic stem cell transplants.
- Melanoma survivors are at higher risk for other skin cancers (even for another melanoma) later in life.
- Brittle nails are more common in women, the elderly, people whose hands get wet frequently, and those who had chemotherapy or stem cell transplants.
- Persistent hair loss (more than six months after treatment) is more common in people who had transplants or chemotherapy with busulfan, carboplatin, cyclophosphamide, docetaxel, paclitaxel, or thiotepa.
- Guidelines for transplant survivors can be found at the Center for International Blood and Marrow Transplant Research (CIBMTR) website: www.cibmtr.org.
- Around 15 percent of all survivors will have lymphedema; risk factors include an initial cancer of the breast, genitals, or head, as well as melanomas, sarcomas, obesity, and treatments that required surgery and radiation.
- For soft-tissue cancers, radiation therapy can be given before or after surgery. When given before surgery, there are more wound complications, but fewer long-term effects, such as skin swelling and fibrosis.

one third of survivors who have had chemotherapy report still having skin, hair, or nail conditions six months after the end of treatment. Here are some of the side effects that may occur and ways to manage them.

Dark Skin Discoloration

Skin darkening can result from a number of different medicines that either directly stimulate skin color (pigment) formation or cause a rash that, when healed,

> **DID YOU KNOW?**
>
> The most common skin problems experienced by survivors include persistent hair thinning, scars, skin cancers, and lymphedema.

Sun and Survivors: Playing It Safe

Because the sun's ultraviolet rays are a major cause of skin cancer, aging, burns, and discoloration, it's important for survivors to protect themselves by using a broad-spectrum sunscreen with a sun protection factor (SPF) of at least 15. Avoid sun exposure between 10 am and 4 pm, and wear protective clothing and sunglasses. (For more details, see Chapter 10, "Sun Safety.") *Survivors should have yearly skin checkups by a trained professional to make sure there are no suspicious growths, a potential warning sign for skin cancer.*

Fortunately, about two thirds of survivors report using sunscreen; even more use sunscreen if they've received radiation therapy. Survivors (especially women and those with lighter skin) are also less likely to sunbathe or use tanning beds than are other people.

DID YOU KNOW?

Most people don't realize that fluorescent lights emit small amounts of ultraviolet rays. In fact, eight hours under a fluorescent lamp is equivalent to one minute in the sun. So it's a good idea to use sunscreen, even when indoors.

leaves darker spots (or red spots, in fair-skinned people). The latter is a skin's defense mechanism known as post-inflammatory hyperpigmentation, in which any type of rash or skin bump heals by leaving dark-colored spots.

If darkening occurs, it's important to avoid sun exposure or exposure to indoor fluorescent lights, without sunscreen protection.

Treatments for skin darkening include creams such as tretinoin, azelaic acid, or the bleaching cream hydroquinone. But the most important first treatment is, of course, prevention or early treatment. Whatever the cause, darkening may last for months to years, so it can be frustrating to many people. But there are steps that you and your doctor can take to improve this side effect. If creams do not work, a dermatologist or plastic surgeon may be able to help with special procedures, such as peels or lasers.

White Skin Discoloration

White spots or skin lightening can also occur as a side effect of some medications, especially all-trans-retinoic acid, arsenic trioxide, lenalidomide, imatinib, interferon, ipilimumab, pazopanib, and sunitinib. Whitening is usually reversible; the skin can go back to normal several weeks or even months after the culprit medications are stopped.

There are other conditions that may occur during treatment with anti-cancer medications that cause skin lightening: a yeast infection called tinea versicolor results in whitish dry spots on the upper chest and back; vitiligo causes large white areas on the face and hands; and pityriasis alba causes whitish oval spots on the face and body of children. In addition, graft-versus-host disease (GVHD) can also result in white skin discoloration, which can last for many months or even years. All of these conditions can be differentiated from those caused by anti-cancer medications, and most of them can be treated with topical medications, including anti-fungals or corticosteroids.

Although there is no safe way to stimulate skin color in an effort to correct skin lightening, there are effective ways to conceal these color changes. Foundations and concealers are available in tints that match just about any skin color. The brands Cover FX and Amazing Cosmetics are two examples.

Red Skin Discoloration

Redness usually results once a rash has healed, especially in fair-skinned people.

A common problem is the post-inflammatory redness that occurs after a bumpy or acne-like rash has faded. Usually, this is seen on the face or chest when drugs such as cetuximab, docetaxel, erlotinib, gefitinib, paclitaxel, or panitumumab, have been used. The redness (or erythema, as doctors call it) can last for many months if not treated. Treatment includes topical medicines that shrink the blood vessels (oxymetazoline). Another way to deal with redness is to have a dermatologist or plastic surgeon use a special laser on the skin.

DID YOU KNOW?

When radiation is used after surgery, surgical wounds heal better than when radiation is given before the procedure, but there is a higher chance of skin swelling and hardening.

I finished my chemotherapy, so can I take vitamins or supplements to improve the appearance of my skin, and should I get some sun to keep my vitamin D levels high?

 Before taking any vitamin or supplement, tell your oncologist, since they may interfere with other medications. Approximately 80 percent of survivors take vitamin or mineral supplements, with 30 percent starting to use them after their diagnosis. The American Cancer Society (ACS) recommends taking a standard multivitamin/mineral supplement containing 100 percent of the recommended daily allowance. The ACS discourages the use of high-dose supplements. Through a simple blood test, your doctor can check your levels of vitamin D, which should be at least 30 ng/mL. Sun exposure is not recommended as a means of increasing vitamin D, since it is easily available in supplements. Finally, antioxidants (such as vitamin E and beta-carotene) have not been shown to improve the skin's appearance or texture.

DID YOU KNOW?

Beta-carotene supplements should be avoided, especially by smokers. Prostate cancer survivors have to avoid calcium and zinc supplements in particular. Those who have or have had colon cancer should avoid folic acid supplements.

Hair Changes (Thinning, Changes in Texture)

For most people who lose their hair during treatment, it will grow back. Hair color or texture in about one third of people may grow back differently: those with straight hair may find their hair grows in curly (the so-called chemo curls). On the other hand, those who had curly hair may grow it straight. Hair color can also change: dark hair may grow back gray, whereas light hair may grow back darker, although that is more unusual. It's not known exactly how many people who have lost their hair from chemotherapy will not grow back a full head of hair. Usually, two months after the end of chemotherapy, hair starts growing again. It tends to grow about half an inch every month, or about five inches a year. The speed of hair growth varies, depending on genetics, gender, and age. Normal hair growth after chemotherapy may be affected by other factors such as weight loss, anemia (low levels of red blood cells), or deficiencies in biotin (a vitamin) or zinc (a mineral). Hormones or other blood-related changes (menopause, thyroid disease, low levels of iron and vitamin D) can also slow hair growth.

Some survivors do experience hair thinning or loss lasting more than six months after chemotherapy. Persistent hair loss is more common in people who received busulfan and stem cell transplants or chemotherapy with carboplatin, cyclophosphamide, docetaxel, paclitaxel, or thiotepa. The good news is that this is usually caused by most hairs being at continued rest, which means that there are things that can be done to "get them going." Your doctor can check your blood for underlying causes, such as an underactive thyroid, altered levels of male-female hormones, and a decreased amount of vitamin D and ferritin (which stores iron in the blood and is recommended at levels above 70 for women who have hair loss). Your doctors can prescribe medications to adjust these levels. I also recommend using minoxidil 5% twice daily on the scalp and supplements of biotin (2.5 mg or 2,500 mcg a day) and orthosilicic acid 10 mg a day (BioSil, two tablets daily).

While things are getting back to normal, consider using a wig, hair extensions, or hair thickeners (diCesare Thicken Hair Builder, DermMatch Topical Shading, or Toppik Hair Building Fibers). Sprays and powders can also cover the scalp (Top Coverage for Bald Spot and Thinning Hair, Bumble and Bumble Hair Powder). These products give the appearance of a fuller head of hair. Most of these products are available in different colors (gray, blonde, brown, and black).

> **DID YOU KNOW?**
>
> In a survey of cancer survivors, dry skin, itching, and nail changes were the most common side effects that had a negative impact on their lives during treatment.

Nail Changes (Darkening, Brittle, or Slow Growing)

Anti-cancer medications can have lingering effects on the nails, hands, or feet (resulting in dry, thick areas in the palms and soles). In a survey, nail problems were the second most common unexpected side effect that affected cancer survivors.

Nail discoloration (dark or purple color) can be caused by bleomycin, capecitabine, cyclophosphamide, dacarbazine, daunorubicin, docetaxel, doxorubicin, fluorouracil, idarubicin, imatinib, methotrexate, paclitaxel, sorafenib, sunitinib, topotecan, and vincristine. Eventually, nails will grow, and the color will go back to normal. In the meantime, you can stimulate your nails to grow faster by taking biotin and orthosilicic acid supplements or hide the discoloration by applying a dark-colored nail polish. Some dark, chemical-free nail polishes include OPI Lincoln Park after Dark or Black Cherry Chutney, China Glaze Evening Seduction, Sally Hansen Pat on the Black, Polished Mama Date Night.

Nails are 15 percent water but can get dryer when they split and during the winter. So be especially careful during these times. It's common for nails to become brittle as a result of treatment. Perhaps it's not surprising, since nails are flattened skin cells that become very hard (similar to claws in animals). So when anti-cancer medications slow down or block the growth of the skin, nails are also affected. It's important to note that women's nails are thinner and more brittle than men's nails.

Fingernails grow very slowly (about one tenth of an inch every month), so if chemotherapy makes them brittle, they will remain that way for some time: it takes about six months to grow a fingernail and about one year to grow a toenail (as we age, nails grow more slowly). Brittle nails are not a trivial condition; when nails are healthy and hard, they protect the tip of the finger, enhance sensitivity of the fingertips, and sometimes act as tools to grasp tiny things. When brittle nails break, they can hurt, making it uncomfortable to perform simple everyday tasks.

Brittle nails are also associated with thyroid, kidney, and liver diseases, which your doctor can diagnose with a blood test. So how can you avoid brittle nails? Take biotin and orthosilicic acid, and apply a nail strengthener every day. Remember that just getting your nails wet with detergents, nail polish removers, or even water makes them more likely to become brittle. If these measures don't help, your dermatologist may prescribe a vitamin A cream (tazarotene), that when applied twice daily to nails will make them

stronger. Nail hardeners with up to two percent formalin may also provide an additional benefit. Apply two
topcoats after applying nail polish and one coat of nail
strengthener daily (CITRA Formaldehyde-Free #3; OPI
Nail Envy Natural Nail Strengthener; China Glaze Nail
Strengthener & Growth Formula; Sally Hansen Hard As
Nails strengthener).

If nails are thick and yellow after chemotherapy,
it is possible that a fungal infection has occurred. This
happens especially in people who had chemotherapies
that affect the nails, such as capecitabine, cetuximab,
docetaxel, doxorubicin, erlotinib, lapatinib, paclitaxel,
and panitumumab. Your doctor may take a sample of
your nail to confirm this and may recommend treatment with oral or topical antifungal medications. If
only a few nails are affected, laser treatment can also
be done to destroy nail fungus by an experienced podiatrist or a dermatologist.

Surviving Surgery

Almost all cancer survivors have had some procedure
or surgery as part of their cancer diagnosis or treatment. Scars, lymphedema, and amputation are the
most common results of surgery. We'll discuss each of
those in turn here.

Scars

Unless problem scars are treated, they will not improve
with time. Most cancer survivors are unaware of treatments for problem scars, even though there are many
ways to improve them. Studies in childhood cancer survivors have shown that up to 25 percent have scars on
the head and neck, 18 percent on the arms and legs,
and up to 38 percent on the chest and stomach. These
scars, especially on the head and neck, can affect people
emotionally and affect their quality of life—but doctors
can reduce the size, pain, tightness, and appearance of
these scars. Sometimes, just one type of treatment can
significantly improve the look of a scar. In other cases,

a combination of approaches may offer the best results. Consult with your dermatologist or plastic surgeon to find the right treatment for you.

The hallmarks of problem scars are that they grow too big and are larger than normal; itch or hurt; are unsightly or embarrassing; and feel tight or limit the movement of the neck, arm, leg, or other body part. For all of these issues, usually something can be done—your doctor may prescribe silicone gel sheets to be applied over the scar, corticosteroid creams, adhesive tapes, or injections. Laser treatments, medical tattooing, or microdermabrasion at a dermatologist or plastic surgeon's office may also be appropriate if the initial treatments don't work. You can even have a procedure, called a scar revision, to "re-create" the scar. For more information on scar treatments, see Chapter 8, "Your Skin After Surgery."

Lymphedema

When a cancer surgeon removes a number of lymph nodes, in the armpit or groin area, for example, a side effect that can show up well after the surgery is lymphedema. This condition is marked by an abnormal swelling of an arm or leg. The tissues of the limbs swell because lymphatic fluid builds up and cannot drain into the now-

Q I have lymphedema on my left arm after surgery for breast cancer. I like working out, including lifting some weights. Can I exercise with my arm?

A For many years, people were told that they could not lift objects with their lymphedema-affected arm. Now we know that exercise, including weight lifting, can actually decrease lymphedema, probably because the muscles squeeze the fluid out of the arm or leg. Therefore, exercise is not only allowed but encouraged, especially since obesity is a proven risk factor for lymphedema. If you are using a compression sleeve, you can keep using it during exercise. As always, it's best if a certified physical therapist supervises your exercise program.

Lymphedema Do's and Don'ts

By working with your doctor and a lymphedema therapist and following the measures described below, you can regain a sense of control and reduce symptoms.

- Get fitted for a compression garment.
- Have regular manual lymphatic drainage by a therapist.
- Avoid having injections or blood pressure measurements in your affected arm.
- Take good care of your skin, keeping it clean and moisturized.
- If you cut or break the skin in an area where you have had lymphedema, apply Polysporin ointment twice daily.
- If you have had lymph nodes removed from the underarm area, use an electric hair trimmer if you wish to remove hair under your arm. Avoid close shaves or waxing.
- When getting a manicure, make sure instruments are sterilized. If possible, avoid cutting the cuticles; it's better just to push them back.
- When outdoors, use an insect repellent spray or OFF! Clip-On Mosquito Repellent.
- Use protective gloves when washing dishes, gardening, or cleaning.
- Remove jewelry or tight-fitting clothing that leave a mark.
- Do not use hot water or heating pads on the area.
- Avoid sunburn by using a broad-spectrum sunscreen with an SPF of at least 15 or protective clothing.

removed lymph nodes. Lymph nodes are small, bean-shaped organs found throughout the body, that play an important role in removing waste and fluids, helping to fight off infections. An area swollen with lymphedema feels heavy, tender, and tired, and the skin may feel tight.

After surgery, people susceptible to lymphedema usually notice it for the first time if they sustain an injury (such as a burn) or an infection, after strenuous activity, weight gain, or flying on an airplane. If this happens to you, it is important to notify your doctor right away, especially if there is any redness and pain, which may indicate an infection that requires oral antibiotics (such as cephalexin or trimethoprim-sulfamethoxazole).

With a procedure called sentinel lymph node biopsy, the risk of developing lymphedema has been reduced to 10 percent. In this procedure, only one lymph node is removed during surgery (the node into which cancer cells are most likely to spread). If many or all of the lymph nodes in the area being treated are removed during surgery, 20 to 30 percent of people will develop lymphedema. Radiation, infections, being overweight, burns, or injuries in the area of surgery can also increase the risk. Swelling can begin a few weeks after surgery and last for many years if not treated properly. This includes caring for the skin in the affected area as well as keeping the area elevated, getting lymphatic massages, and using compression garments. For more information, see Chapter 8, "Your Skin After Surgery."

Amputation

For cancers of the bones or soft tissues (such as sarcomas), in the arms or legs, amputation is frequently performed as a cure. Although it is a significant procedure, people with amputations may report a better quality of life than those who have large surgeries that do not involve amputation—the so-called limb-sparing operations. In these limb-sparing surgeries, artificial bones or joints are sometimes placed in the body, which may end up requiring additional complicated procedures. That is why doctors may suggest amputation as an option. Many people with amputations, either with or without a prosthesis (an attachable limb), say they adjust as well as other people, with no greater anxiety, depression, or loss of self-esteem. Long-term amputation survivors can live full and productive lives.

In some cases, amputations are necessary because of infections that develop in a surgical area. It's important to work with a physical medicine and rehabilitation doctor or a dermatologist if you experience any skin side effects after an amputation.

Skin Effects of Amputation

- Blisters, redness, or bruising from a poorly fitting prosthesis (artificial limb)
- Shooting pains, severe cramping, or a burning sensation
- Skin breakdown and slow healing of the remaining wound
- Emotional distress related to a change in body image

It is important to take good care of your skin in the amputated limb, especially in the areas that come into contact with the prosthesis. The area should be kept clean and dry, with special attention to spots that change color. Make sure that the washable items (such as the stump shrinker, elastic garments, stump socks) are washed with a gentle, fragrance-free detergent. For young people who are still growing, the prosthesis has to be evaluated by a prosthetist every six months and then once yearly after they stop growing. If at any point the prosthesis is hurting, or blisters appear in the area, the prosthetist should be notified. In the meantime, it is a good idea to apply the topical antibiotic Polysporin to prevent any infections.

DID YOU KNOW?

Areas of skin that received radiation do not heal as well as those that did not. So if you are having any type of surgical procedure in a previously radiated area, make sure you tell your surgeon.

Surviving Radiation Therapy

Almost half of all cancer survivors have received radiation therapy during their treatment. Most people experienced the immediate effects of radiation (skin redness, swelling, itching, and pain). However, these side effects usually go away several weeks after the end of radiation therapy. But some changes may persist well after radiation therapy has finished.

- Skin darkening
- Dilated, red blood vessels
- Hardening or tightness of the skin
- Loss of hair, sweat, and oil glands, leading to persistent hair thinning or loss and dry skin that doesn't sweat

Addressing the After-Effects of Radiation

Symptom	What Can Be Done To Improve It
Skin darkening	Bleaching creams (hydroquinone), lasers, or chemical peels
Dilated blood vessels (redness)	Laser treatment
Dry, flaky skin	Exfoliant (ammonium lactate, lactic acid, or salicylic acid creams)
Skin fibrosis	Vitamin E plus pentoxifylline orally, topical corticosteroids, physical therapy
Hair thinning or loss	Minoxidil, biotin, orthosilicic acid
Slow nail growth	Biotin, orthosilicic acid
Wounds or sores that do not heal	Evaluation by a dermatologist or wound specialist. Important to rule out infections and skin cancer, as they can look like wounds.
Growths, skin cancers	Evaluation by a dermatologist to rule out skin cancer. Skin cancers are usually surgically removed. Benign (non-cancerous) growths can also be removed if they cause pain or discomfort.
Dry mouth	Artificial saliva sprays (Mouth Kote, Biotene), gels or liquids (Optimoist, Biotene Oral Balance, Numoisyn) or lozenges (Numoisyn, up to 14 a day), saliva stimulants such as cevimeline (30-mg tablets three times a day) or pilocarpine (5-mg tablets three times a day). Consider acupuncture, if all else fails.
Radiation tattoos	Laser or surgical removal

Lasers, peels, and other skin procedures should be performed by a plastic surgeon or dermatologist.

- Slow nail growth or nail loss (can occur if radiation was given close to the tips of the fingers or toes)
- Wounds that don't heal, and scars that are inflamed
- Skin cancers or growths, which usually appear three years or more after radiation therapy

- Dry mouth, if radiation was given to the face or neck area

The chronic effects of radiation depend on the total dose of radiation as well as the amount given at each session (also called "fraction"). Skin is most affected when more than 200 centigray (cGy) is given at each fraction. Radiation techniques have improved considerably, so people who received radiation in the past 30 years are at a lower risk for persistent skin changes. Areas of radiation can have slower hair growth as well as less sweating, causing the skin to be drier. Persistent hair thinning or loss after radiation therapy depends on how much radiation was given. If less than 1,800 cGy of radiation was given, hair growth is usually normal; more than that amount may result in permanent hair thinning. This will be more noticeable in survivors who received radiation for cancers on the head. For permanently thin or lost hair, an evaluation by a dermatologist or plastic surgeon with experience in hair loss and hair transplants is advisable. For more information, visit the website of the International Society of Hair Restoration Surgery (www.ishrs.org).

Although cancerous tissues are its intended target, radiation can destroy other tissues, so it's not surprising that in certain cases, the skin heals by forming a scar. Just as with a scar that forms after a cut, the skin is tight, shiny, sometimes itchy, and of a different color. Unlike a scar from a cut, which is usually a line, a radiation-induced scar is usually spread out across the entire area of skin that received radiation. In some cases, the scar goes deeper into the skin. This type of scarring is called fibrosis. For people who received radiation for cancers of the neck, breast, and rectum, fibrosis is common. An evaluation by a physical medicine and rehabilitation doctor (physiatrist) would be very helpful. They may recommend certain exercises guided by a physical therapist, injections into tight muscles, and anti-inflammatory creams for areas that are sore or tight. For people who have decreased sweating, it is

DID YOU KNOW?

Tattooing by an experienced professional can significantly help scars that are associated with skin color changes or hair loss, such as on the face, eyebrow, scalp, or any other area.

important to avoid overheating when working out or when temperatures are high. Using a moisturizer regularly is also key, since the glands that produce skin oils will usually be decreased. More information on skin changes after radiation therapy is available in Chapter 7, "Side Effects of Radiation Therapy."

Surviving Stem Cell Transplants

As a cancer survivor, the most important condition to be aware of after a bone marrow or stem cell transplant is GVHD. This is discussed further in Chapter 9, "Stem Cell Transplants and Your Skin."

The acute form of GVHD usually occurs within the first three months after treatment and results in a red, bumpy skin rash. Doctors have made remarkable advances in preventing and treating acute GVHD. Chronic GVHD occurs in 40 to 70 percent of people. The risk of chronic GVHD depends on many factors such as where the stem cells where obtained from, the degree of match between donor and recipient, and the use of anti-GVHD medications. Chronic GVHD usually develops from six months to two years after the transplant. However, it can appear years and sometimes even decades later. For people who haven't developed chronic GVHD by the second or third year after treatment, the chances become lower over time. At the five-year mark, only about 20 percent of people are on medications to treat chronic GVHD.

Skin affected by GVHD can present in many different ways. It can look like a red, bumpy rash, with spots of many different shapes and sizes. The skin may be darker, along with some hardening or tightening. Flaking or dryness is also common, especially on the scalp and upper body.

It is important to notify your doctor as soon as any sign of GVHD appears, to prevent the symptoms from becoming worse, or any discomfort. In most cases, the symptoms of chronic GVHD improve with treatment.

How chronic GVHD is treated depends on its severity: for grade 1 (mild), when less than one fifth

Chronic GVHD: What to Look For

- Dryness or flaking, especially on the scalp, face, and upper body
- Dark or whitish spots anywhere on the body
- Hardness, tightness, dimpling, or thinning of the skin
- Decreased sweating and dry mouth
- Dilated blood vessels in the skin (looking like big veins)
- Difficulty moving joints or opening the mouth from tight skin
- Whitish or red spots or sores in the mouth or on the genitals
- Hair thinning, dullness, or graying
- Brittleness or ridging of the nails or nail loss

of the skin's surface is affected by rash or hard/tight skin, your doctor may prescribe topical medications (fluocinonide, or tacrolimus). For grade 2 (moderate) GVHD, in which up to half of the skin on the body is affected, the addition of oral medications to suppress the immune system is usually needed (prednisone, sirolimus, or tacrolimus, among others). In grade 3 (severe) chronic GVHD, when more than half of the skin is involved, oral medicines may need to be combined with external treatments such as UV light treatments at a dermatologist's office (phototherapy) or extracorporeal photopheresis (treating the blood with drugs activated by UV light). If you take oral immunosuppressive medicines, your doctor may also prescribe oral antibiotics, anti-virals, and anti-fungals, to prevent infections.

DID YOU KNOW?

Cancer survivors who have received radiation may develop dilated blood vessels or skin tightness, which can be improved with laser treatments, oral medicines, and physical therapy, respectively.

For chronic GVHD in the mouth, if the white areas and/or sores do not affect eating, treatment is usually started with topical medicines four times a day. They include either a medicated paste (triamcinolone in orabase) for localized sores or a mouthwash (dexamethasone solution) when the areas are widespread. When using topical corticosteroids in the mouth, it's always a good idea also to dissolve an antifungal lozenge

DID YOU KNOW?

Chronic GVHD usually needs to be treated in order to prevent limitation of function and serious infections.

(clotrimazole) four times a day in the mouth, to prevent commonly occurring fungal infections. If GVHD in the mouth becomes severe enough to affect eating, your doctor may prescribe the oral immunosuppressive medicines previously listed or add numbing medicines to the mouthwash (lidocaine gel or mouthwash). For dry or chapped lips, hydrocortisone (Cortizone-10, Hytone) or tacrolimus ointment applied three times a day usually helps. Avoid licking your lips, since saliva irritates the skin. If there is vaginal irritation or dryness, the same approach can be taken (Cortizone-10, Hytone) or tacrolimus ointment applied three times a day, but always consult with a gynecologist or dermatologist specializing in genital conditions.

In chronic GVHD, flaky and dry areas often appear on the scalp, neck, and face. Although this may look like simple dryness, it usually represents a lingering inflammation (similar to when you get a sunburn and the skin starts peeling off). Therefore, moisturizers alone usually are not enough. Topical corticosteroids and exfoliants work the best. For dry, flaky areas on the scalp, use the following daily: corticosteroid shampoos (clobetasol, fluocinolone), solutions (clobetasol or fluocinonide), or foams (clobetasol, betamethasone). On the face, hydrocortisone (Hytone) or tacrolimus ointment twice daily will help. If scaling or dryness persists on the face, using a face wash containing a low concentration of salicylic acid will help (Neutrogena Oil-Free Acne Wash Salicylic Acid Acne Treatment, Olay Acne Control Face Wash). As always, avoid face scrubs and astringents, which may irritate your skin even more.

For most people who have had transplants, the hair and nails look and feel normal afterward. In a small number of people, the hair may be thin, dull, and brittle. The nails may also grow more slowly and have grooves. For care of hair and nails after transplant, follow the same guidelines as in Chapter 9, "Stem Cell Transplants and Your Skin." Recommended supplements for stronger and faster growth of both nails and hair are biotin

(Appearex 2.5 mg or 2,500 mcg a day) and orthosilicic acid 10 mg a day (BioSil, 1 capsule twice daily).

In summary, stem cell transplants are an effective treatment for many cancers of the blood, and many people remain cured. But knowing what to expect years after the transplant can greatly improve the ability to live well. The chemotherapy received as part of the preparation, the type of transplant, and the time since the transplant will affect the development of skin conditions. Other than dry and thinning skin, most people will not even notice any skin changes after their transplants. The risk of skin cancer is higher in transplant survivors, especially if radiation was used, so having yearly skin checks by your doctor or dermatologist is important. Make sure to tell them if you notice any changing mole or spot on your skin.

> **DID YOU KNOW?**
> Only 1 out of 10 cancer survivors visit a dermatologist during treatment; if you don't have a dermatologist already caring for your skin, now is the time to see this type of specialist.

If You Are a Childhood Cancer Survivor

People younger than age 21 who have been diagnosed with cancer have a very good chance of being completely cured of their disease. Recently, it has been found that survivors of childhood cancers need to be monitored closely, as treatment early in their lives can have long-term effects on their overall health, especially when it comes to the skin, heart, kidneys, teeth, bones, liver, breasts (in women), and immune system. Guidelines created by doctors and the Children's Oncology Group detail the various conditions that need to be followed and treated so they have the least impact on cancer survivors' lives. Survivorship guidelines for the long-term follow-up of childhood, adolescent, and young adult cancers are an important resource of the Children's Oncology Group, available at www.survivorshipguidelines.org.

When it comes to long-term changes in skin and hair, most childhood cancer survivors would benefit from extra care. But it turns out that only half of cancer survivors see a dermatologist for their skin problems,

Childhood Cancer Survivors: What Are the (Skin) Risks?

Dermatologic Issue	Types of Treatment and/or Childhood Cancer
Persistent hair thinning	Acute lymphoblastic leukemia (ALL)
	Acute myeloid leukemia (AML)
	Brain tumors
	Radiation therapy
Skin cancers in areas of radiation	Acute myeloid leukemia (AML)
	Brain tumors
	Hodgkin lymphoma (HL)
	Neuroblastoma
	Non-Hodgkin lymphoma (NHL)
	Sarcomas (including Ewing's sarcoma and osteosarcoma)
	Wilms tumor
Problem scars	Neuroblastoma
	Sarcomas (including Ewing's sarcoma and osteosarcoma)
	Surgery, port placement
	Wilms tumor
Dry mouth	Hodgkin lymphoma (HL)
Dark skin discoloration	Chemotherapy with bleomycin, daunorubicin, doxorubicin, etoposide, and idarubicin
	Radiation therapy
	Stem cell transplants
Stretch marks	Corticosteroids (prednisone, dexamethasone)
Melanoma	Certain testicular cancers

such as skin cancers, hair loss, scars, and nail fungal infections. This highlights the importance of yearly skin examinations (especially those who received radiation therapy, or chemotherapy with etoposide or teniposide), since their skin cancers occur earlier (at about age 30) than in other people (over 50 years of age).

The most common type of skin cancer in survivors is called basal cell carcinoma, the most benign type of all. Usually, a local procedure is all that is needed to cure it. The risk for skin cancers is higher in cancer survivors who were treated with radiation, especially before the age of 20. Since radiation therapy for many childhood cancers usually involves the scalp, it's important for yearly skin exams to include the scalp, even under the hair. Hairdressers can be very helpful in looking for and pointing out any new or changing spots on the scalp that may need to be evaluated by a dermatologist.

There are good reasons for childhood cancer survivors to involve a dermatologist in their care; they include stretch marks, scars, and hair thinning. Stretch marks occur especially in children who received corticosteroids as part of their treatment for brain cancers or during stem cell transplants. Although difficult to treat, stretch marks in cancer survivors may be improved with the use of topical medications (tretinoin, tazarotene) or peels and laser treatments by a dermatologist or plastic surgeon. Scars from surgery and radiation are common in children, especially on the chest or stomach (in 30 percent), head or neck (25 percent), or arms and legs (18 percent). In addition, hair loss occurs in 14 percent of childhood cancer survivors, mostly in those who received high doses of radiation to the brain. All of these conditions can negatively affect survivors' quality of life, so every effort to minimize them with the help of a dermatologist can go a long way in making life better.

> **DID YOU KNOW?**
>
> Tinted foundations or creams can be used to conceal skin changes caused by cancer treatments.

Tips for Cancer Survivors

Reducing the chances of skin cancers is very important, especially in people who have received radiation therapy or transplants.

Other than sunscreen and creams containing vitamin A (tretinoin, tazarotene), there are no vitamins, supplements, or antioxidants that prevent skin cancers or minimize skin aging.

Resources

Children's Oncology Group Long-Term Follow-Up Guidelines for Survivors of Childhood, Adolescent, and Young Adult Cancers	www.survivorshipguidelines.org
National Lymphedema Network	www.lymphnet.org (800) 541-3259
American Cancer Society	www.cancer.org (800) 227-2345
Cancer Information Service	www.cancer.gov (800) 422-3762
Amputee Coalition	www.amputee-coalition.org (888) 267-5669
National Coalition for Cancer Survivorship	www.canceradvocacy.org (877) 622-7937
Let's Face It (for people with facial differences)	desica.dent.umich.edu/faceit/
Locks of Love	www.locksoflove.org (888) 896-1588
Beyond the Cure	www.beyondthecure.org (800) 5-FAMILY
Center for International Blood and Marrow Transplant Research	www.cibmtr.org (414) 805-0700
ACOR's Site for Families of Survivors of Childhood Cancer	www.ped-onc.org/survivors/

Not all skin changes after treatment are of concern; chemotherapy and radiation therapy increase the number of benign (non-cancerous) moles in childhood caner survivors.

For brittle nails, avoid frequent exposure to water and nail polish removers and use a moisturizer after hand washing. Keep your nails short, trim them horizontally after showering, and when filing, do it in one direction. Taking biotin and orthosilicic acid (BioSil) and applying nail strengtheners every day are also helpful.

Hair loss that persists after chemotherapy or radiation therapy is not common. After excluding other causes of hair loss, you can use camouflaging methods (wigs, sprays, or powders), oral vitamins and supplements, and topical hair stimulators (minoxidil).

Transplant survivors should be especially careful with sun exposure, since their risk of skin cancer is greater. Also, certain medications taken after a transplant heighten the risk for sensitivity to the sun (such as trimethoprim/sulfamethoxazole and voriconazole).

If dryness, itching, or rash develops any time after a stem cell transplant, it is important to notify your doctor. They can be signs of GVHD. Tell your doctor if you have had any eye, mouth, genital, or gastrointestinal changes, as they may be associated with GVHD.

Keep the area with lymphedema elevated (for example an arm should rest on pillows above the level of your heart). Use a compression garment as directed by a lymphedema therapist or doctor, especially when traveling by airplane. Exercise is allowed and recommended.

Physical medicine and rehabilitation doctors (also called physiatrists or rehab medicine doctors) are invaluable in helping with many of the side effects affecting cancer survivors, ranging from difficulty moving joints to lymphedema, tight skin, amputations, and more.

Keep a copy of your medical records and a list of all your medications (prescription, natural products, supplements, vitamins, over-the-counter) with you. Give this list to your health care provider (doctor, nurse, etc.) every time you have an appointment. Wear an allergy ID bracelet or necklace (www.americanmedical-id.com, www.medicalert.org, www.laurenshope.com) for special medical issues or if you have any allergies.

THINGS TO REMEMBER

- Childhood cancer survivors need special attention paid to their skin, especially if they have received radiation therapy. Their skin must be examined by a health care provider at least once a year.

- Hair thinning can persist after chemotherapy or radiation therapy, but it is rare. To find the cause, factors such as thyroid hormone, vitamin D, and iron levels may need to be checked.

- Most cancer survivors say that dry skin and irritation were some of the most bothersome side effects resulting from their treatment. Moisturizers and gentle soaps should reduce these issues significantly.

- Twenty percent of people have brittle nails (women and the elderly are twice as likely to be affected), and this is even more frequent in people after stem cell transplants.

- Most survivors of stem cell transplants have skin that is more sensitive to dryness, irritation, and the sun.

- Problem scars from surgeries or ports can usually be improved with topical or injectable medications or minor surgical procedures performed by a dermatologist or plastic surgeon.

- Lymphedema is a chronic condition, so it is important always to continue with follow-ups and recommendations from your lymphedema therapist and/or doctor. Be sure to inform them of any changes.

- Physical medicine and rehabilitation doctors have the tools and knowledge to improve cancer survivors' function and ability to perform daily routines that involve the physical, psychological, social, and vocational aspects of life.

- People who have had amputations should notify their prosthetist if the prosthesis breaks; new noises appear in the area (popping, squeaking, etc.); you have outgrown the prosthesis; or you have chronic pain while wearing the prosthesis.

- Dermatologists are important allies in the overall care of cancer survivors: by performing skin checks and improving scars, brittle nails, hair thinning, or any other skin condition.

Appendix A:
Skin, Hair, and Nail Side Effects
of Anti-Cancer Medications

Use this table to look up potential side effects of the medications you are taking for treating your cancer. This information has been obtained from each medication's prescribing information and from published scientific medical literature.

Generic name / *Brand name*	Use	Potential side effects (skin; hair; nail)
Abarelix / *Plenaxis*	Prostate cancer	Hot flashes, breast enlargement, nipple tenderness, leg swelling
Abiraterone / *Zytiga*	Prostate cancer	Leg swelling, hot flashes
Alemtuzumab / *Campath*	Leukemia, lymphoma	Allergic reactions, face swelling, blistering, infections, itching, cold sores, shingles, leg swelling, purple spots, welts, rash, sweating, lip and mouth sores
All-trans retinoic acid (ATRA) / *Vesanoid*	Leukemia	Worsening acne, rash, blistering, skin irritation, severe dryness, infections, sweating, facial and leg swelling, sensitivity to sunlight, itching, dry mouth, lip and mouth sores; Hair thinning; Painful swelling of nail folds
Altretamine / *Hexalen*	Ovarian cancer	Rash, itching; Hair thinning
Anastrozole / *Arimidex*	Breast cancer	Hot flashes, face swelling, sweating, leg swelling, itching, rash, dry mouth, vaginal dryness; Hair thinning
Asparaginase / *Elspar, Erwinaze*	Leukemia	Allergic reactions, face swelling, sweating, leg swelling, rash, itching, blistering, welts, lip and mouth sores
Arsenic trioxide / *Trisenox*	Leukemia	Rash, itching, hot flashes, purple spots and discoloration, dryness, redness, sweating, face swelling, white or dark discoloration, welts, cold sores or shingles, pain at site of injection, dry mouth
Axitinib / *Inlyta*	Kidney cancer	Hand-foot syndrome, dry skin, redness, itching, mouth sores; Hair thinning
Azacitidine / *Vidaza, Mylosar*	Myelodysplastic syndrome	Injection site redness or reaction, dry skin, itching, purple skin discoloration, rash, welts, mouth sores

Generic name / *Brand name*	Use	Potential side effects (skin; hair; nail)
Bevacizumab / *Avastin*	Various cancers	Rash, sores, dryness, nosebleeds, poor wound healing, mouth sores and taste changes
Bendamustine / *Treanda*	Leukemia, lymphoma	Allergic reactions, rash, purple skin discoloration, itching, dry skin, sweating, cold sores or shingles, dry and sore mouth
Bexarotene / *Targretin*	Lymphoma	Acne, infections, rash, face swelling, irritation, sores, leg swelling, sensitivity to sunlight, itching, blistering, dryness, dry mouth; Hair thinning
Bicalutamide / *Casodex*	Prostate cancer	Hot flashes, sweating, swelling, rash, shingles, itching, dryness, dry mouth, breast enlargement (in men); Hair thinning
Bleomycin / *Blenoxane*	Lymphoma, head and neck, genital, and testicular cancers	Allergic reactions, face swelling, blistering, rash, redness, red or dark lines, dark discoloration, itching, painful sensitivity to cold in fingers and toes, hardening, welts, stretch marks, lip and mouth sores; Hair loss, graying; Nail horizontal ridges or dark bands, brittleness, loss, slow growth
Brentuximab vedotin / *Adcetris*	Lymphoma	Rash, itching, dry skin, blisters, sweating, leg swelling; Hair thinning
Bortezomib / *Velcade*	Multiple myeloma, lymphoma	Rash, blisters and sores, shingles, leg swelling
Busulfan / *Busulfex, Myleran*	Leukemia, stem cell transplant preparation	Darkening of the skin, dryness, welts, itching, dry mouth, lip sores; Hair thinning
Cabazitaxel / *Jevtana*	Prostate cancer	Mouth sores, leg swelling; Hair loss; Nail color changes or loss
Capecitabine / *Xeloda*	Breast and colorectal cancers	Hand-foot syndrome, rash, precancers in skin, rash in previously sunburned or radiated areas, sensitivity to sunlight, dark discoloration, itching, dryness, sores, lip and mouth sores; Hair thinning; Brittleness, nail loss, separation, inflammation in nail folds, thickening under nails
Carboplatin / *Paraplatin*	Lung and ovarian cancers	Allergic reactions, mouth sores; Hair loss
Carmustine / *BiCNU*	Brain cancer, lymphoma, multiple myeloma	Rash, redness, dark discoloration or burns if contacts with skin, pain or burning in area of injection
Cetuximab / *Erbitux*	Colorectal and head/neck cancers	Acne-like rash, dryness, cracks in fingertips and heels, itching, sensitivity to sunlight, redness, allergic reactions, infections; Hair thinning and curling on scalp and body, increased growth and thickening of hair on the face, long and curly eyelashes; Painful inflammation in nail folds, slower growth, brittleness
Chlorambucil / *Leukeran*	Leukemia, lymphoma	Allergic reactions, rash, blisters
Cisplatin / *Platinol*	Lung, ovarian, and testicular cancers, lymphoma, sarcomas	Allergic reactions, rash; Hair loss

Generic name / *Brand name*	Use	Potential side effects (skin; hair; nail)
Cladribine / *Leustatin*	Leukemia	Allergic reactions, sweating, swelling, infection, redness, rash, shingles, itching, purple spots, blistering, welts, pain at site of injection
Clofarabine / *Clolar*	Leukemia	Rash, itching, redness, hand-foot syndrome, cold sores or shingles, swelling, skin infections, mouth sores
Crizotinib / *Xalkori*	Lung cancer	Mouth sores, rash
Cyclophospha-mide / *Cytoxan*	Lymphoma, leukemia, neuroblastoma, retinoblastoma, ovarian and breast cancers	Allergic reactions, rash; Hair loss; Nail horizontal lines or ridges, brittleness, white or dark discoloration
Cytarabine (Ara-C) / *Cytosar-U*	Leukemia	Allergic reactions; rash; purple spots; welts; shingles; itching; blistering; lip, mouth, and anal sores; Hair thinning
Dacarbazine / *DTIC, DTIC-Dome*	Melanoma, lymphoma	Swelling, face redness, sensitivity to sunlight, welts; Hair thinning
Dactinomycin (actinomycin D) / *Cosmegen*	Testicular, uterine cancers, sarcomas, Wilms and Ew-ing's tumors	Acne, blistering, infection, rash in previously radiated areas, dark discoloration, pain at site of injection, lip and mouth sores; Hair loss
Dalteparin / *Fragmin*	Blood clots (prevention or treatment)	Allergic reactions, face swelling, rash, itching, purple spots, blistering, sores, welts, pain or rash or bumps at site of injec-tion; Hair thinning
Darbepoetin alfa / *Aranesp*	Low levels of red blood cells (anemia)	Allergic reactions, itching, rash, infections, swelling, welts, red-ness, mouth sores, pain at site of injection
Dasatinib / *Sprycel*	Leukemia	Rash, sensitivity to light, dark discoloration, itching, welts, dry-ness, sores, lip and mouth sores; Hair thinning; Brittleness
Daunorubicin / *Cerubidine*	Leukemia	Swelling, rash, itching, welts, pain at site of injection, lip and mouth sores; Hair loss
Decitabine / *Dacogen*	Myelodysplas-tic syndromes	Purple or white skin discoloration, rash, itching, welts, face and leg swelling, mouth sores, bleeding; Hair thinning
Degarelix / *Degarelix for injection*	Prostate cancer	Inflammation at site of injection, hot flashes, enlargement and tenderness of breasts (in men)
Denileukin diftitox / *Ontak*	Lymphoma	Allergic reactions, rash, sweating, itching, swelling, inflamma-tion at site of injection
Docetaxel / *Taxotere*	Breast, head and neck, prostate, and stomach cancers	Allergic reactions, dryness, leg swelling, redness, hand-foot syndrome, rash in previously sunburned or radiated areas, itching, purple spots, rash, hardening, blistering, welts, lip and mouth sores; Hair loss (reversible in most people); Nail hori-zontal ridges, brittleness, nail loss, white or dark discoloration, painful inflammation of folds, separation of nails, thickening, painful infections, bleeding under nails

Generic name / *Brand name*	Use	Potential side effects (skin; hair; nail)
Doxorubicin / *Adriamycin, Caelyx, Doxil, Rubex*	Various cancers, leukemia, lymphoma, multiple myeloma	Hand-foot syndrome, allergic reactions, swelling, infections, blistering, rash in folds, dryness (especially in palms and soles), sores, rash in previously sunburned or radiated areas, itching, welts, dark spots in lips and tongue, lip and mouth sores; Hair loss; Nail horizontal ridges or white lines, dark vertical lines
Eculizumab / *Soliris*	Diseases of red blood cells	Cold sores, pain in extremities
Eltrombopag / *Promacta*	Few platelets in the blood	Purple spots
Enoxaparin / *Lovenox*	Blood clots (prevention or treatment)	Allergic reactions, rash, itching, purple spots, blistering, sores, welts, pain or rash or bumps at site of injection
Epirubicin / *Ellence*	Breast cancer	Rash, itching, mouth sores; Hair loss
Epoetin alfa / *Epogen, Procrit*	Low levels of red blood cells (anemia)	Allergic reactions, itching, rash, welts; Hair thinning, increased hair growth on face
Eribulin / *Halaven*	Breast cancer	Mouth sores; Hair loss; Nail color changes, infections, loss
Erlotinib / *Tarceva*	Lung and pancreatic cancers	Acne-like rash, dryness, cracks in fingertips and heels, itching, sensitivity to light, redness, infections; Hair thinning and curling on scalp and body, increased growth and thickening of hair on the face, long and curly eyelashes; Painful inflammation in nail folds, slower growth, brittleness
Estramustine / *Emcyt, Estracyt*	Prostate cancer	Allergic reactions, face swelling or hot flashes, rash, dark discoloration, itching, dryness, purple spots, welts, dryness, breast tenderness or enlargement, sweating, pain at site of injection; Hair thinning
Etoposide / *Eposin, VePesid, VP-16*	Lung and testicular cancers	Allergic reactions, sweating, redness, blistering, rash in previously sunburned areas, itching, dark discoloration, purple spots, welts, lip and mouth sores; Hair loss; Nail horizontal lines or ridges
Everolimus / *Afinitor*	Kidney, pancreatic, and brain cancers	Rash, itching, dryness, lip and mouth sores and dryness, swelling; Nails brittle, loss, or pain and infections in folds
Exemestane / *Aromasin*	Breast cancer	Hot flashes, sweating, leg swelling, itching, rash; Hair thinning
Filgrastim / *Neupogen*	Bone marrow transplants, low levels of white blood cells	Painful sores, allergic reactions, rash, itching, welts, pain or bumps at sites of injection
Floxuridine / *FUDR*	Colorectal and stomach cancers	Rash, mouth sores; Hair thinning
Fludarabine / *Fludara*	Leukemia, stem cell transplant preparation	Swelling, rash, purple spots, lip and mouth sores, skin cancers, metallic taste; Hair thinning
Fluorouracil / *Adrucil*	Colon, breast, and pancreatic cancers	Dry skin, sensitivity to sunlight, dark skin discoloration along veins, rash, hand-foot syndrome, rash, swelling, lip and mouth sores; Hair loss

Generic name / *Brand name*	Use	Potential side effects (skin; hair; nail)
Fluoxymesterone / *Halotestin*	Breast cancer	Acne, rash, swelling, itching, dandruff; Hair thinning, increased hair growth on face
Flutamide / *Eulexin*	Prostate cancer	Hot flashes, pain at site of injection, breast enlargement and pain (in men)
Fondaparinux / *Arixtra*	Blood clots (prevention or treatment)	Allergic reactions, rash, itching, purple spots, bleeding into the skin, blistering, sores, welts, pain or rash or bumps at site of injection
Fulvestrant / *Faslodex*	Breast cancer	Hot flashes, sweating, leg swelling, rash, pain at site of injection
Gefitinib / *Iressa*	Lung cancer	Acne-like rash, dryness, cracks in fingertips and heels, itching, sensitivity to sunlight, redness, infections; Hair thinning and curling on scalp and body, increased growth and thickening of hair on the face, long and curly eyelashes; Painful inflammation in nail folds, slower growth, brittleness
Gemcitabine / *Gemzar*	Various cancers	Allergic reactions; areas that are painful, swollen, and red, especially on the legs; rash in previously radiated areas; painful sensitivity to cold in fingertips; pain at site of injection; lip and mouth sores; Hair thinning or loss
Goserelin / *Zoladex*	Breast and prostate cancers	Hot flashes, allergic reactions, swelling, rash, welts, vaginal dryness, sweating, dandruff, discoloration, acne, breast enlargement and pain (in men), pain or bumps at site of injection; Hair thinning
Hydroxyurea / *Hydrea*	Leukemia, melanoma, ovarian and head and neck cancers	Rash, sores, darkening, purple spots, swelling, redness, dryness, skin cancer, mouth sores; Hair thinning; Brittle nails
Ibritumomab / *Zevalin*	Lymphoma	Allergic reactions, sweating, blistering, sweating, leg swelling, purple spots, rash, itching
Idarubicin / *Idamycin, Zavedos*	Leukemia	Hand-foot syndrome, blistering, welts, rash in previously radiated areas, welts, rash at site of injection, lip and mouth sores; Hair loss; Dark nail discoloration
Ifosfamide / *Ifex, Ifosfamidum*	Testicular and various other cancers	Allergic reactions, blisters, hand foot syndrome, redness, rash in radiated sites, purple spots, sweating, sores, darkening; Hair loss; Ridges
Imatinib / *Gleevec*	Leukemia, sarcoma, gastrointestinal and blood cancers	Rash, skin cancers, swelling, redness, sores, white or dark discoloration, dryness, purple spots, blistering, sensitivity to sunlight, itching, lip or mouth sores, welts; Hair thinning; Nail brittleness, dark discoloration
Interferon alfa / *Infergen, Intron A*	Melanoma, leukemia, and lymphoma	Allergic reactions, rash, sweating, itching, purple spots, painful sensitivity to cold in fingers and toes, welts, white discoloration, pain at site of injection; Hair thinning, darkening, increased hair on face and eyelashes, change in texture
Interleukin-2 (aldesleukin) / *Proleukin*	Kidney cancer, melanoma	Allergic reactions, blistering, rash, cold sores, shingles, leg swelling, itching, purple spots, welts, pain at site of injection, lip and mouth sores; Hair loss
Ipilimumab / *Yervoy*	Melanoma	Rash, itching, white skin discoloration; Hair and eyelash graying or whitening

Generic name / *Brand name*	Use	Potential side effects (skin; hair; nail)
Irinotecan (CPT-11) / *Camptosar*	Colorectal cancer	Allergic reactions, sweating, rash, lip and mouth sores; Hair loss
Ixabepilone / *Ixempra*	Breast cancer	Hand-foot syndrome, rash, itching, dark discoloration, blisters, hot flashes, allergic reactions; lip and mouth sores; Hair thinning; Dark or white nail discoloration, nail separation and loss
L-Asparaginase / *Elspar*	Leukemia	Allergic reactions
Lapatinib / *Tykerb*	Breast cancer	Rash, dry skin, itching, redness, mouth sores; Hair thinning; Painful inflammation in nail folds, slower growth, brittleness
Lenalidomide / *Revlimid*	Multiple myeloma, myelodysplastic sydromes	Rash, sweating, redness, leg swelling, itching, dryness, purple spots, nosebleeds, infections, dry mouth, lip and mouth sores
Letrozole / *Femara*	Breast cancer	Hot flashes, sweating, rash, leg swelling, itching, blistering; Hair thinning
Leucovorin / *Fusilev*	Osteosarcoma, colorectal cancer, anemias, and when methotrexate or fluorouracil is used	Mouth sores, rash; Hair thinning
Leuprolide / *Lupron, Viadur*	Prostate cancer	Hot flashes, acne, rash, sweating, leg swelling, sensitivity to sunlight, breast enlargement and pain (in men), bumps or pain at sites of injection, taste changes, vaginal inflammation; Hair thinning
Lomustine, CCNU / *Ceenu*	Brain cancers, lymphoma	Mouth sores; Hair thinning
Mechlorethamine / *Mustargen*	Lymphoma, leukemia, lung cancer	Allergic reactions, welts, blisters, shingles, rash; Hair loss
Medroxyprogesterone / *Prempro, Provera*	Endometrial and breast cancers	Acne, allergic reactions, face swelling, dark discoloration of face, sweating, rash, itching, hardening, stretch marks, welts, hot flashes, breast enlargement and pain (in men); Hair thinning, increased hair growth on face
Megestrol / *Megace*	Breast and endometrial cancers, appetite stimulant	Acne, rash, itching, sweating, breast enlargement (in men), cold sores; Hair thinning
Melphalan / *Alkeran*	Myeloma, ovarian cancer, stem cell transplant preparation	Allergic reactions, rash; Hair loss; Nail discoloration
Mercaptopurine / *Purinethol*	Leukemia	Rash, dark discoloration, mouth infections; Hair thinning

Generic name / *Brand name*	Use	Potential side effects (skin; hair; nail)
Methotrexate / *Abitrexate, Folex, Mexate*	Leukemia, lymphoma, breast, lung, endometrial, bone, and head and neck cancers	Acne, redness, blistering, cold sores and shingles, hair follicle infections and inflammation, rash in areas of previous sunburn or radiation, sensitivity to sunlight, itching, dark discoloration, skin sores, welts, lip and mouth sores, purple spots; Hair thinning
Mitomycin / *Mutamycin*	Stomach and pancreatic cancers	Rash, pain, and inflammation at injection site, redness or sores in the skin, lip and mouth sores, purple spots; Hair loss
Mitotane / *Lysodren*	Adrenal gland cancer	Rash, purple spots, lip and mouth sores, breast enlargement and pain (in men)
Mitoxantrone / *Novantrone*	Leukemia, prostate cancer	Allergic reactions, lip and mouth sores, purple spots, swelling, sweating, welts, pain and inflammation at the site of injection; Hair loss
Nelarabine / *Arranon*	Leukemia and lymphoma	Purple discoloration, lip and mouth sores, leg swelling
Nilotinib / *Tasigna*	Leukemia	Itching, rash, leg swelling, eyelid swelling, sweating, welts, purple spots, sensitivity to sunlight, skin discoloration, dryness; Hair thinning
Nilutamide / *Nilandron*	Prostate cancer	Hot flashes, sweating, swelling, itching, rash, dryness, breast enlargement and pain (in men), dry mouth; Hair thinning
Octreotide / *Sandostatin*	Carcinoid and VIP tumors	Allergic reactions, swelling, welts, breast enlargement (in men), pain at site of injection; Hair thinning
Ofatumumab / *Arzerra*	Leukemia	Rash, welts, sweating, shingles, leg swelling, allergic reactions
Oprelvekin / *Neumega*	Bleeding (low level of platelets)	Allergic reactions, swelling, rash, discoloration, mouth infections
Oxaliplatin / *Eloxatin*	Colorectal cancer	Allergic reactions, nosebleeds, mouth sores, leg swelling, rash; Hair thinning
Paclitaxel / *Abraxane, Taxol*	Breast, lung, ovarian cancers, Kaposi's sarcoma	Allergic reactions, rash, dryness, leg swelling, hand-foot syndrome, rash in previously radiated areas, lip and mouth sores, pain at site of injection, tightness; Hair loss (reversible in most patients); White or dark discoloration or bands, painful inflammation of folds, separation of nails, thickening
Panitumumab / *Vectibix*	Colorectal cancer	Acne-like rash, dryness, cracks in fingertips and heels, itching, sensitivity to sunlight, redness, allergic reactions, infections; Hair thinning and curling on scalp and body, increased growth and thickening of hair on face, long and curly eyelashes; Painful inflammation in nail folds, slower growth, brittleness
Pazopanib / *Votrient*	Kidney cancer	Rash, face swelling, hand-foot syndrome, white discoloration, dryness, lip and mouth sores; Hair thinning, graying
Pegaspargase / *Oncaspar*	Leukemia	Rash, hives, itching, leg swelling, rash at sites of injection
Pegfilgrastim / *Neulasta*	Bone marrow transplants, low level of white blood cells	Acne, cysts, painful sores, allergic reactions, sweating, swelling, redness, rash, itching, welts, pain or bumps at site of injection, taste change, lip and mouth sores; Hair loss

Generic name / *Brand name*	Use	Potential side effects (skin; hair; nail)
Pemetrexed / *Alimta*	Lung cancer, mesothelioma	Allergic reactions, peeling, swelling, rash in previously sun-burned areas, sores in areas of pressure, itching, purple spots, leg swelling, lip and mouth sores
Pentostatin / *Nipent*	Leukemia, graft-vs-host disease	Rash, mouth sores, shingles, skin infection
Plerixafor / *Mozobil*	Lymphoma, multiple myeloma	Inflammation at the site of injection
Porfimer sodium / *Photofrin*	Esophageal, lung cancers	Sensitivity to sunlight, rash, itching
Pralatrexate / *Folotyn*	Lymphoma	Mouth sores, rash, swelling
Procarbazine / *Matulane*	Lymphoma, brain cancer	Allergic reactions, rash, cold sores and shingles, dark discoloration, itching, purple spots, redness, welts, lip and mouth sores; Hair thinning
Raloxifene / *Evista*	Osteoporosis, breast cancer	Hot flashes, sweating, leg swelling, rash, vaginal inflammation
Rituximab / *Rituxan*	Lymphoma	Allergic reactions, face swelling, rash, sweating, blistering, shingles, leg swelling, itching, welts, pain at site of injection, lip and mouth sores
Romidepsin / *Istodax*	Lymphomas of the skin	Rash, itching, swelling, lip and mouth sores
Sipuleucel-T / *Provenge*	Prostate cancer	Allergic reactions
Sargramostim / *Leukine*	After bone marrow transplants, low level of white blood cells	Rash, pain and inflammation at site of injection
Sorafenib / *Nexavar*	Kidney and liver cancers	Hand-foot syndrome, acne, moles, growths and cancers, dryness, redness, welts, scalp pain, nipple tenderness, itching, lip and mouth sores; Hair thinning and curling; Dark vertical lines in nails
Streptozocin / *Zanosar*	Pancreatic cancer	Purple spots, pain and inflammation at area of injection
Sunitinib / *Sutent*	Kidney and gastrointestinal cancers	Hand-foot syndrome, leg swelling, yellow discoloration, dandruff-like rash, dryness, eyelid swelling; Hair thinning, graying; Dark vertical lines in nails
Tamoxifen / *Nolvadex*	Breast cancer	Swelling, hot flashes, sweating, rash, dryness; Hair thinning, increased hair on face, hair darkening
Temozolomide / *Temodar*	Brain cancer, melanoma	Allergic reactions, swelling, dry skin, itching, rash, lip and mouth sores; Hair thinning
Temsirolimus / *Torisel*	Kidney cancer	Allergic reactions, lip and mouth sores, rash, itching, infections, dry skin, acne, swelling; Nail inflammation
Teniposide / *Vumon*	Leukemia, lymphoma, lung cancer	Allergic reactions, allergic reactions, rash, welts, lip and mouth sores, purple spots; Hair loss

Generic name / *Brand name*	Use	Potential side effects (skin; hair; nail)
Thalidomide / *Thalomid*	Multiple myeloma	Rash, allergic reactions, swelling, itching, purple spots, lip and mouth sores, dryness; Hair thinning; Brittle nails
Tioguanine / *Lanvis*	Leukemia	Purple spots, dry mouth, lip and mouth sores; Hair loss
Thiotepa / *Thioplex*	Before stem cell transplants, some breast, ovarian, bladder cancers	Allergic reactions, rash; Hair loss
Tinzaparin / *Innohep*	Blood clots (prevention or treatment)	Allergic reactions, purple spots, pain or rash or bumps at site of injection
Topotecan / *Hycamtin*	Ovarian, cervical, and lung cancers	Rash, purple spots, lip and mouth sores; Hair loss
Toremifene / *Fareston*	Breast cancer	Hot flashes, sweating, swelling, dark discoloration, rash; Hair thinning
Tositumomab / *Bexxar*	Lymphoma	Allergic reactions, swelling, sweating, itching, rash
Trastuzumab / *Herceptin*	Breast, stomach cancers	Acne, allergic reactions, leg swelling, rash; Hair thinning; Brittle nails
Vandetanib / *Caprelsa*	Thyroid cancer	Rash, acne, rash, dry skin, dark spots, itching
Vemurafenib / *Zelboraf*	Melanoma	Rash, dry skin, itching, moles, hand-foot syndrome, growths and skin cancers; Hair thinning and curling
Vinblastine / *Velban, Velsar*	Lymphoma, endometrial, breast, Kaposi sarcoma, and testicular cancers	Rash, blistering, sensitivity to sunlight, lip and mouth sores; Hair loss
Vincristine / *Oncovin, Vincasar*	Leukemia, lymphoma, spinal cord and muscle, and kidney tumors	Allergic reactions, rash; Hair loss
Vinorelbine / *Navelbine*	Lung and breast cancers	Allergic reactions, pain at site of injection; Hair loss
Vismodegib / *Erivedge*	Advanced basal cell cancer	Rash, dry skin, loss of taste; Hair thinning
Vorinostat / *Zolinza*	Skin lymphoma	Leg swelling, itching, rash; Hair thinning
Warfarin / *Coumadin*	Blood clots (prevention or treatment)	Allergic reactions, rash, purple spots, sores, itching, welts; Hair thinning

Appendix B:
List of Anti-Cancer Medications by Brand Name

Use this table to look up the generic name of the medication you are taking by its brand name. If you do not see the brand name of your medication listed here, please ask your oncologist.

Brand Name	Generic Name	Brand Name	Generic Name
Abitrexate	Methotrexate	Busulfex	Busulfan
Abraxane	Paclitaxel	Caelyx	Doxorubicin
Adcetris	Brentuximab vedotin	Campath	Alemtuzumab
Adriamycin	Doxorubicin	Camptosar	Irinotecan (CPT-11)
Adrucil	Fluorouracil	Caprelsa	Vandetanib
Afinitor	Everolimus	Casodex	Bicalutamide
Alimta	Pemetrexed	CeeNU	Lomustine, CCNU
Alkeran	Melphalan	Cerubidine	Daunorubicin
Aranesp	Darbepoetin alfa	Clolar	Clofarabine
Arimidex	Anastrozole	Cosmegen	Dactinomycin (actinomycin D)
Arixtra	Fondaparinux	Coumadin	Warfarin
Aromasin	Exemestane	Cytosar-U	Cytarabine (Ara-C)
Arranon	Nelarabine	Cytoxan	Cyclophosphamide
Arzerra	Ofatumumab	Dacogen	Decitabine
Avastin	Bevacizumab	Doxil	Doxorubicin
BiCNU	Carmustine	DTIC, DTIC-Dome	Dacarbazine
Bexxar	Tositumomab	Ellence	Epirubicin
Blenoxane	Bleomycin	Eloxatin	Oxaliplatin

Brand Name	Generic Name	Brand Name	Generic Name
Elspar	L-Asparaginase	*Intron A*	Interferon alfa
Emcyt	Estramustine	*Iressa*	Gefitinib
Epogen	Epoetin alfa	*Istodax*	Romidepsin
Eposin	Etoposide	*Ixempra*	Ixabepilone
Erbitux	Cetuximab	*Jevtana*	Cabazitaxel
Erivedge	Vismodegib	*Lanvis*	Tioguanine
Erwinaze	Asparaginase	*Leukeran*	Chlorambucil
Estracyt	Estramustine	*Leukine*	Sargramostim
Eulexin	Flutamide	*Leustatin*	Cladribine
Evista	Raloxifene	*Lovenox*	Enoxaparin
Fareston	Toremifene	*Lupron*	Leuprolide
Faslodex	Fulvestrant	*Lysodren*	Mitotane
Femara	Letrozole	*Matulane*	Procarbazine
Firmagon	Degarelix	*Megace*	Megestrol
Fludara	Fludarabine	*Mexate*	Methotrexate
Folex	Methotrexate	*Mozobil*	Plerixafor
Folotyn	Pralatrexate	*Mustargen*	Mechlorethamine
Fragmin	Dalteparin	*Mutamycin*	Mitomycin
FUDR	Floxuridine	*Myleran*	Busulfan
Fusilev	Leucovorin	*Mylosar*	Azacitidine
Gemzar	Gemcitabine	*Navelbine*	Vinorelbine
Gleevec	Imatinib	*Neulasta*	Pegfilgrastim
Halaven	Eribulin	*Neumega*	Oprelvekin
Halotestin	Fluoxymesterone	*Neupogen*	Filgrastim
Herceptin	Trastuzumab	*Nexavar*	Sorafenib
Hexalen	Altretamine	*Nilandron*	Nilutamide
Hycamtin	Topotecan	*Nipent*	Pentostatin
Hydrea	Hydroxyurea	*Nolvadex*	Tamoxifen
Idamycin	Idarubicin	*Novantrone*	Mitoxantrone
Ifex	Ifosfamide	*Oncaspar*	Pegaspargase
Ifosfamidum	Ifosfamide	*Oncovin*	Vincristine
Infergen	Interferon alfa	*Ontak*	Denileukin diftitox
Inlyta	Axitinib	*Paraplatin*	Carboplatin
Innohep	Tinzaparin	*Photofrin*	Porfimer sodium

Brand Name	Generic Name	Brand Name	Generic Name
Platinol	Cisplatin	*Treanda*	Bendamustine
Plenaxis	Abarelix	*Trisenox*	Arsenic trioxide
Prempro	Medroxyprogesterone	*Tykerb*	Lapatinib
Procrit	Epoetin alfa	*Vectibix*	Panitumumab
Proleukin	Interleukin-2 (aldesleukin)	*Velban*	Vinblastine
Promacta	Eltrombopag	*Velcade*	Bortezomib
Provenge	Sipuleucel-T	*Velsar*	Vinblastine
Provera	Medroxyprogesterone	*VePesid*	Etoposide
Purinethol	Mercaptopurine	*Vesanoid*	All-trans retinoic acid (ATRA)
Revlimid	Lenalidomide	*Viadur*	Leuprolide
Rituxan	Rituximab	*Vidaza*	Azacitidine
Rubex	Doxorubicin	*Vincasar*	Vincristine
Sandostatin	Octreotide	*Votrient*	Pazopanib
Soliris	Eculizumab	*VP-16*	Etoposide
Sprycel	Dasatinib	*Vumon*	Teniposide
Sutent	Sunitinib	*Xalkori*	Crizotinib
Tarceva	Erlotinib	*Xeloda*	Capecitabine
Targretin	Bexarotene	*Yervoy*	Ipilimumab
Tasigna	Nilotinib	*Zanosar*	Streptozocin
Taxol	Paclitaxel	*Zavedos*	Idarubicin
Taxotere	Docetaxel	*Zelboraf*	Vemurafenib
Temodar	Temozolomide	*Zevalin*	Ibritumomab
Thalomid	Thalidomide	*Zoladex*	Goserelin
Thioplex	Thiotepa	*Zolinza*	Vorinostat
Torisel	Temsirolimus	*Zytiga*	Abiraterone

Appendix C: Glossary

acne Condition in which oil glands within hair follicles become plugged, causing red or pus-filled bumps. Usually face, chest, and upper back are affected.

acneiform Descriptive term used for any rash that may look like acne but is caused by chemotherapy or other medication.

adverse event (AE) Is the medical term for any undesired or inadvertent condition or disease associated with the use of a medical treatment or procedure, that occurs during the course of treatment.

allergens Substances that cause an allergic reaction. Can be foods (such as eggs, shellfish, fish, nuts), medicines (antibiotics, anti-pain, anti-seizure medicines, chemotherapies), or commonly used ingredients (fragrances, botanicals, preservatives).

allergic contact dermatitis, allergic rash A rash that appears after coming in contact with a substance the body reacts to. Any substance can cause an allergy, even years after having used it. After cancer treatments (chemotherapy, radiation therapy, or surgery), people may develop allergies to things they were never allergic to before.

alopecia Loss of hair, especially on the head. Chemotherapy can cause a loss of body hair, eyebrows, and eyelashes.

ammonia Liquid used in hair bleaches and permanent wave products. May cause hair breakage and irritation to the eyes and mouth. May lead to skin cancer when used at very high doses.

anaphylaxis (also called **anaphylactic shock**) The most severe form of an allergy, in which there is difficulty breathing; abdominal pain; swelling of the eyelids, lips, or tongue; drowsiness or fainting; and dangerously low blood pressure. Fortunately, it is very rare.

anesthetic Numbing medications that can be used topically for itchy or painful areas. Examples are lidocaine, benzocaine, and tetracaine, and their effect usually lasts several hours. Excessive use can lead to allergies or absorption into the body, causing side effects.

angioedema Swelling of the lips or eyelids, usually part of an allergic reaction.

anti-emetic A medication that is effective against vomiting and nausea.

A
B
C

antihistamine Medications used against itching and allergies. Whereas the most effective ones (diphenhydramine and hydroxyzine) can cause drowsiness, others can be taken during the daytime with few side effects (cetirizine, fexofenadine, and loratadine). People with glaucoma and men with a large prostate should use antihistamines with caution.

anti-neoplastic A type of treatment intended to prevent the growth of a tumor or cancer.

aromatase inhibitor (AI) A type of medication that blocks estrogen, used in post-menopausal women with breast or ovarian cancer.

atrophic scar Depressed, soft scar that appears as a dimple on the skin.

avobenzone Also known as Parsol 1789, Eusolex 9020. It's a chemical-based sun-screen that absorbs ultraviolet A. Can be degraded by sunlight, so needs to be combined with another product and applied repeatedly.

azelaic acid Product used against acne or to lighten dark skin spots. Available in creams or gels.

balsam of peru A pleasant-smelling liquid used in many skin and hair products and perfumes. Common cause of allergies or skin irritation.

barrier ingredients Added to creams or ointments to act as a shield against infec-tions and irritation. Common barrier ingredients include petrolatum, paraf-fin, beeswax, and zinc oxide.

benign Not malignant or cancerous. Benign conditions are not dangerous to health.

benzalkonium chloride Antiseptic used in many skin, eye, and hair products. Can be irritating. For safety, skin products should have a concentration no greater than 0.1 percent, whereas hair products can have up to 3 percent.

benzoyl peroxide Antibacterial used in anti-acne creams, gels, and washes. Also dries skin and can bleach or discolor clothing if not rinsed off.

biologic therapy, or biotherapy Medications that help the immune system fight cancer. Some of these drugs are also used to reduce certain side effects.

biotin Vitamin B_7, often used to help nails and hair grow faster and stronger.

body surface area The extent of skin affected by a certain condition, such as a rash. A person's palm is approximately 1 percent of the total skin surface, or body surface area.

bone marrow The spongy tissue inside the bones where blood cells are formed. The marrow contains a large number of stem cells.

broad-spectrum sunscreen The ideal type of sunscreen. It protects against both types of harmful UV-A and UV-B rays from the sun.

calamine A mixture of zinc and ferric oxide often used to relieve itch.

cancer Any malignant growth or tumor caused by abnormal and uncontrolled cell division. After cancer has established itself, it may spread to other parts of the body through the lymphatic system or the bloodstream.

capsaicin Ingredient obtained from hot peppers that is used in creams or oint-ments against itching or pain. Needs to be applied at least four times a day and may temporarily sting or burn when first applied.

cellulitis A spreading infection of the deep tissues of the skin and muscle that usually occurs in the legs, areas with lymphedema, or in a wound after sur-gery. The skin is red, painful, swollen and may be associated with chills and fever.

cheilitis Inflammation of the lips, marked by chapping, redness, cracking, and pain. Causes can be certain types of chemotherapy, radiation, sun, and any type of lipstick, cream, or balm. Licking the lips can also cause cheilitis or make it worse.

chemical peel A method in which a strong chemical is applied for a short period to improve the feel and appearance of scars.

chemotherapy (chemo) Medications given by mouth or through a vein that destroy cancer cells.

chlorhexidine Antiseptic used in many products, available as a wash to cleanse the skin when it is prone to infections. Should not be used on the face, eyes, or ears.

cold cream Cream made from a combination of mineral oil, beeswax, water, and rose petals.

collagen The "glue" that holds the body together, this protein supports the tissues of the skin, bone, and muscles.

comedogenic Any ingredient that causes acne by blocking oil glands in the follicles and creating red or pus bumps and cysts.

concealer A type of facial makeup that hides dark circles, small imperfections, fine lines and wrinkles, and signs of fatigue.

conditioning regimen High doses of chemotherapy, radiation, or both used before a stem cell transplant to improve the chances of success. During this period, people are more susceptible to infections and other conditions, so close observation by the transplant team in the hospital is mandatory.

corticosteroids Available for topical, oral, and intravenous use, these medications reduce inflammation and are effective against many types of rash and allergies. They are also used to help relieve itch.

cosmeceutical A cosmetic that has or claims to have medicinal properties.

cream A white, thick liquid used to moisturize, protect, and deliver medications topically onto the skin. Usually an equal mixture of oil and water, it is easy to spread and does not leave a greasy feel.

cryosurgery A surgical procedure that uses extremely cold liquid to freeze and destroy skin growths. Can be slightly uncomfortable at first; the area treated blisters, scabs, and then falls off.

cutaneous Relating to the skin.

cyst A deep round growth in the skin that can be tender or painful. It is considered benign, or non-cancerous.

debulking The surgical removal of part of a cancer that cannot be completely cut away. Debulking increases the effectiveness of radiation therapy or chemotherapy.

DEET Acronym for diethyltoluamide, a chemical used in insect repellents. Has not been associated with any type of cancer.

dehiscence When a wound reopens or comes apart after it has been surgically closed, due to an infection or other complication.

depilatories Products used to remove hair. Chemical depilatories are very irritating and in most cases should be avoided when receiving chemotherapy. There are wax-based depilatories that may be less irritating.

dermabrasion A surgical method used to improve the feel and appearance of the skin by wearing off the outer layer. It is done using lasers, sandpaper, or other mechanical procedure.

dermatologic Of or relating to the skin, hair, and nails.

dermatologic adverse events, or side effects Any of more than 52 conditions affecting the skin, hair, and nails during cancer treatment with chemotherapy, radiation therapy, or surgery.

desensitization A process in which small and increasing doses of a medication are given to prevent an allergic reaction.

dibutyl phthalate A substance found in nail polish. Listed by California Proposition 65 as a cancer-causing substance. Certain nail polish brands do not use dibutyl phthalate: OPI, China Glaze, Sally Hansen, Zoya, Polished Mama, and Shellac.

dihydroxyacetone (DHA) Coloring ingredient used in artificial or "fake" tanners. Considered safe by the U.S. Food and Drug Administration.

dimethicone A substance used in a variety of products, including shampoos. Does not irritate the skin and is considered safe.

DMDM hydantoin A preservative, reviewed by the Cosmetic Ingredient Review Panel and deemed safe.

donor lymphocyte infusion Sometimes after a stem cell transplant, more stem cells from the donor are given, to produce a greater anticancer effect. This can also trigger graft-versus-hort disease.

dry skin Called "xerosis" by doctors, it is a loss of moisture in the skin.

elastin A protein that coils and recoils like a spring to help keep skin flexible but tight.

electrolysis A permanent hair removal system that uses a needle with a current passed through each hair follicle to destroy the root.

emollient A substance that makes skin soft, supple, and smooth. Can be a lotion, cream, ointment, or spray that coats the dry flakes on the surface of the skin. Petrolatum, zinc oxide, and oils are all emollients.

engraftment The process by which new transplanted stem cells travel to the bone marrow and begin to produce healthy blood cells.

eosinophil A type of cell found in the skin or blood that is usually associated with allergies and itch.

erythema A medical term for redness of the skin.

excoriations A medical term for breaks in the skin caused by scratching.

exfoliant A substance that removes dead skin cells from the top layer of the skin. Ingredients such as ammonium lactate, lactic acid, salicylic acid, and urea are all exfoliants.

external-beam radiation therapy The most common type of radiation treatment in which radiation comes from a machine outside the body.

extravasation The leakage of intravenous drugs from a vein into the surrounding tissue.

foam A preparation used to deliver medications onto hairy areas of the body, such as the scalp. They melt on contact with the skin and are usually available in a can with a nozzle to spray on a cap and then directly onto the skin. Avoid applying on irritated skin.

formaldehyde An irritating preservative used in many cosmetics that can cause allergies. It is used as a preservative in lauryl sulfate, another ingredient used in cosmetics. There have been reports of formaldehyde causing cancer; therefore, it should not be used at a concentration greater than 0.3 percent in non-aerosol cosmetics, except in nail hardeners, where it can be used at a concentration of up to 5 percent.

foundation A skin-colored cosmetic applied to create an even color and to cover rashes, scars, or discoloration. There are four different types: water-based, oil-based, water-free, and oil-free. They can be matched to all types of skin tones.

fragrance-free Cosmetics that are not scented. However, even fragrance-free cosmetics may include substances to mask chemical odors, and they can still cause allergies.

gel A substance used to deliver medicines (a vehicle). Gels are transparent and relatively resistant to being washed off by water. Gels can be drying, irritating, and cause allergies. However, they are good for the scalp and skin folds or for people who don't like a greasy feeling on the skin, since they dissolve upon contact.

grading, or grade The measurement of the severity of a side effect. The grade determines how a side effect is treated and whether anti-cancer treatments should be continued or modified. The most commonly used grading system by doctors is the Common Terminology Criteria for Adverse Events (also known by its acronym, CTCAE).

graft-versus-host disease (GVHD) A condition in which donated stem cells attack the healthy tissues (usually the skin) of the transplant patient. The liver and the intestines can also be affected.

graft-versus-tumor effect The process in which stem cells attack any remaining, cancer cells in the transplant patient. Sometimes the term is more specific based on the underlying type of cancer: graft-versus-leukemia effect, graft-versus-lymphoma effect, or graft-versus-myeloma effect.

growth factors Substances produced by cells that drive their growth. They can also be given by doctors when levels of blood cells become lower than normal.

hair dyes Permanent hair-coloring products. Natural hair dyes contain henna and chamomile. They can result in a more unpredictable color and may not last as long as synthetic hair dyes. Natural dyes can also cause allergies but otherwise are safe. Synthetic dyes can cause skin rashes and irritation.

hirsutism In women, it refers to excess hair growth on the face, where men would normally grow hair.

humectant A substance such as glycerin that absorbs or retains moisture in the skin.

hydrogen peroxide Used in hair bleach preparations for more than 100 years. Can cause burning, redness, or swelling of the scalp.

hydroquinone Bleaching ingredient used in creams for dark discoloration of the skin. Concentrations of more than 2 percent require a prescription from a dermatologist. Four percent is usually the maximum concentration allowed.

hyperkeratosis Thickened, flaky skin that results from the accumulation of dead skin cells on the skin surface. Occurs often in the palms and soles, especially during hand-foot syndrome. The most effective treatments are creams with exfoliants (see definition for **exfoliant**).

hypersensitivity Another name for an allergy, often to a medication.

hypertrichosis Excessive hair growth on any part of the body, applies to both men and women. Can be caused by some medications or diseases.

hypertrophic scars (see also **keloid scars**) Large, abnormal scars that may be disfiguring and associated with itching and pain. They occur most often in the ears, upper chest, and back.

hypoallergenic A term used for products less likely to cause allergies. Some people will still be allergic to these products.

idiopathic Any medical condition or disease with an unknown cause.

idiosyncratic reaction A reaction to a medicine that is unpredictable and usually rare.

immunosuppressive medicines Medications that block the cells in the immune system that are believed to cause graft-versus-hort diseases, allergies, or other diseases mediated by inflammation.

immunotherapy See biologic therapy.

impetigo An infection of the skin usually caused by bacteria. Often seen in people with very dry or itchy skin or in areas of a rash caused by chemotherapy.

inflammation A process in which any part or organ in the body becomes red, swollen, warm, and sometimes even itchy or painful. This may happen as a result of an infection or broken tissue, as the body attempts to repair damage.

intensity-modulated radiation therapy (IMRT) A technique in which radiation is adapted to the shape of the tumor. This technique controls very thin beams of radiation at varying strengths and angles, for a custom-tailored dose that spares healthy tissue and reduces side effects.

intravenous Refers to the method in which a substance, ingredient, or medicine is delivered into the blood through a vein in the arm or a special access port placed under the skin of the chest.

intravesical Administration of chemotherapy through a catheter into the bladder.

keloid scars (see also **hypertrophic scars**) Large, abnormal scars that may be disfiguring and associated with itching and pain. They occur most often in the ears, upper chest, and back.

keratin A strong protein that is an important part of skin, hair, nails, and teeth.

keratosis A benign, non-cancerous skin growth that is usually brown and bumpy. It is easily removed by a dermatologist or plastic surgeon.

lanolin A common ingredient in many moisturizers. It comes from sheep's wool, which some people are allergic to. If you have sensitive skin, avoid lanolin.

laser resurfacing A method used to improve the feel and appearance of the skin or scars through the use of lasers.

lesion A particular change in the skin (a bump or flat area that is unlike normal skin).

lotion A topical preparation that is liquid, used to moisturize or deliver medications onto the skin. Since they are so liquid, they are easy to spread over large or hairy areas of the body.

lumpectomy Surgical removal of a breast lump.

lymph fluid A bodily fluid that circulates throughout the skin and other organs. Lymph picks up microbes or damaged cells and brings them to lymph nodes to be destroyed. Metastatic cancer cells can also be transported via the lymph fluid.

lymph nodes Small, bean-shaped structures throughout the body that help filter out and destroy microbes and damaged cells.

lymphatic system A part of the immune system, which is made up of a network of channels called lymphatic vessels that transport a clear fluid known as lymph (see lymph fluid) to the lymph nodes.

lymphedema Swelling of the skin or a body part after surgery or radiation therapy to the lymph nodes that drain the area.

macule A spot on the skin or a change in the color of the skin.

maculopapular Description of a rash, which is made up of a combination of spots (macules) and bumps (papules). Also termed **morbilliform** (see definition below).

malignant A cancerous growth.

melanonychia Long black or brown streaks in the nails.

moist peeling (or moist desquamation) One of the most severe types of skin reactions to radiation. The skin is red, peeling, moist and frequently is associated with pain and infections, requiring oral antibiotics.

moisturizer A substance that imparts or restores moisture in the skin. Ideally applied several times a day, including within 15 minutes of showering or bathing.

morbilliform rash A common rash caused by many types of medicines, which looks like measles (or looks **maculopapular**, see definition above). The rash appears as red or pink bumps or skin discoloration, especially in the upper body. The rash is usually distributed evenly on the body. Antibiotics, anti-pain, chemotherapies, or anti-seizure medications are common culprits.

mucositis Inflammation of the tissue in the mouth or anal area, associated with sores and pain. Often affects people receiving radiation to the head or neck or anus, stem cell transplants, or certain chemotherapies.

neoadjuvant The use of chemotherapy or radiation before surgery to reduce the size of the cancer, making surgery smaller and more likely to succeed.

neomycin A common antibiotic included in many over-the-counter antibacterial products such as Neosporin or Triple Antibiotic. Many people are allergic to it, so it's best to avoid it.

neurodermatitis A chronic skin disorder associated with severely itchy patches of skin that lead to intense scratching or rubbing and thickening of the skin.

nodule A deep growth or lump in the skin, which could represent an infection or a benign or malignant growth.

non-comedogenic A product or ingredient that does not clog the pores or cause acne.

non-myeloablative transplantation (see also **reduced-intensity transplantation**) The use of lower doses of chemotherapy, with or without radiation, to increase the chance that donated stem cells will become part of the patient. This method usually results in fewer side effects, especially for older people and those with other medical conditions.

non-steroidal anti-inflammatory drugs Also called NSAIDs, they are some of the most commonly used medications to relieve pain, reduce inflammation, and decrease fever. Examples include ibuprofen and naproxen.

ointment A thick, transparent preparation made mostly of oil, in some water. Used as a moisturizer and to deliver certain medications topically. Good for people with dry skin, allergies, or irritation, but many people don't like them because they are so greasy.

onycholysis An often painful separation of the nail from the fingertip, usually caused by chemotherapies. These nails are more susceptible to infections.

onychomycosis A very common fungal infection of the nails, in which the nails become thick and yellow. Fungal infections can develop in nails after they've been affected by chemotherapy or stem cell transplants.

oral Refers to taking a substance, ingredient, or medicine by mouth in the form of a pill, tablet, capsule, or liquid.

papule Small, rounded, raised bump or lesion on the skin.

para-aminobenzoic acid (PABA) An ingredient in sunscreens that used to be included in many different brands. Can cause allergies and discoloration of clothing, so PABA-free sunscreens are recommended today.

parabens A common preservative used in all types of cosmetic and self-care products. There is some concern that it may act like estrogen, so many products no longer use parabens.

paraneoplastic When changes in the skin are found to be linked to cancer, they are called paraneoplastic (from the Greek words *para*, which means alongside, and *neoplasia*, which means new growth). These conditions are quite rare and not well understood. They usually improve or resolve when the underlying cancer is treated.

paronychia Skin infection or inflammation around the nails. Common culprits are the so-called targeted chemotherapies or others such as capecitabine, docetaxel, doxorubicin, and paclitaxel.

petrolatum Also called Vaseline or petroleum jelly. It is made from petroleum and is probably one of the best products to maintain moisture and softness of the skin. Some people may have allergies to it.

phototherapy Treatment in which a light is shone by a special machine at a dermatologist's office, to treat skin diseases such as eczema, rashes, psoriasis, and itching. Also called light therapy, it is sometimes given in combination with oral or topical medications to enhance the effect.

phthalate This chemical and many of its forms are present in many products to soften or dissolve other ingredients. There has been a long-standing concern about this product, so it has been banned in many cosmetics.

pressure sore An open, crater-like sore (or ulcer) on the skin caused by constant pressure or friction, usually from staying in the same position for long periods.

prophylactic or prophylaxis A treatment that is started before a side effect appears, aimed at preventing it. Frequently used to prevent chemotherapy-induced nausea, vomiting, allergies, or rashes.

prurigo Itchy, hard bumps on the skin.

pruritus The medical term for itch. It is the most common and bothersome symptom associated with rashes.

radiation dermatitis A common side effect of radiation treatment. The affected skin becomes painful, red, itchy, and blistered.

radiation recall reaction The development of skin inflammation at a previously radiated site, usually triggered by chemotherapy or other medications.

radiation treatment (also called **radiotherapy** or **irradiation**) High-energy radiation used to kill cancer cells, it can be given using a machine outside the body (external-beam radiation) or with radioactive seeds inside the body planted near the tumor (brachytherapy).

reduced-intensity transplantation (see also **non-myeloablative transplantation**) The use of lower doses of chemotherapy, with or without radiation, to increase the chance that donated stem cells will become part of the patient. This method usually results in fewer side effects, especially for older people and those with other medical conditions.

salicylic acid An exfoliant used in creams to treat inflammation; itch; and dry, flaky, or thick skin. Must be used with caution on irritated skin, as it can sting or burn.

scar revision A surgical procedure used to improve the feel and appearance of scars, usually done by a plastic surgeon.

sebaceous gland A gland that lubricates the hair and the skin. These glands are more abundant on the face, scalp, and the mid and upper chest and back, hence they are called "seborrheic" areas by doctors.

seborrheic dermatitis Medical term for dandruff. Red areas with yellow scales or dry patches that appear on the scalp, chest, and even on the face. Seen more frequently in older people, in those with neurologic disorders, or with the use of certain anti-cancer medicines (sunitinib and temozolomide).

sorbitol Used in creams, lozenges, or liquids to stimulate or replace saliva in cases of dry mouth.

stem cells Immature (or "blank") cells in the blood or bone marrow that can become any type of blood cell: red blood cells carry oxygen, white blood cells fight infection, and platelets control bleeding.

stippling To paint or draw by means of dots or small touches, such as when applying concealer to the face.

subungual hemorrhage Bleeding underneath the nails, which looks like dark streaks. Caused by certain chemotherapies, such as docetaxel, paclitaxel, sorafenib, or sunitinib.

sun protection factor (SPF) The degree to which a sunscreen, suntan lotion, or similar product protects the skin from ultraviolet B rays. An SPF of 10 means that the sunscreen will allow the skin to remain free of redness 10 times longer in the sun than if unprotected by that sunscreen.

Talcum powder Powders containing talc have been linked to ovarian cancer in women who use them on their genitals or groin. Alternatives include powders containing cornstarch.

targeted treatment or therapy A new type of chemotherapy designed to block specific molecules or protein "targets" in cancer cells, stopping their growth and destroying them. These proteins are also necessary for the normal growth of skin, hair, and nails, which explains why so many people develop dermatologic side effects when receiving targeted treatment.

telangiectasias A medical term for dilated or open blood vessels in the skin, which can appear on the face or chest after a rash or radiation treatment. People commonly refer to them as "broken" blood vessels. Can be minimized with lasers by a dermatologist or plastic surgeon.

tolerance The process by which a person becomes less sensitive to a medication, with continued administration. In many cases, this process results in a decrease in the severity of medication-induced rash over time.

toluene sulfonamide/formaldehyde resin Used as a nail strengthener or hardener. Although it has it in the name, this substance does not release any formaldehyde. Some people can be allergic to it or develop skin irritation.

topical Refers to the application of a medicine on the skin. Medicines can be embedded in creams, gels, foams, lotions, ointments, solutions, or sprays.

transplant In oncology, a procedure in which cells from the blood or bone marrow are taken from a healthy person and placed inside a person with certain kinds of cancers of the blood, most commonly leukemias or lymphomas.

trichomegaly Excessive growth of eyelashes and eyebrows.

tumor, or neoplasm A medical term referring to a new growth of any tissue in the body. When this tissue grows uncontrollably, it is called a malignant tumor, or neoplasm.

ultraviolet (UV) rays Part of the invisible light spectrum, primarily found in sunlight. UV rays can damage the skin and affect human health.

urea An exfoliant ingredient used in creams for its ability to moisturize the skin and remove dry, flaky skin. Safe product, but it has a scent and may leave a whitish residue when applied.

urticaria The medical term for hives or welts, usually part of an allergic reaction.

vasoconstriction When blood vessels are reduced in size, due to cold, certain chemotherapies, or topical medicines.

vasodilation When blood vessels are expanded, causing a warm, red sensation. May appear like a hot flash on the face.

xerosis The medical term for dry skin. Dry mouth is termed xerostomia.

zinc oxide A mineral used in sunscreens or in barrier creams. As a sunscreen, zinc oxide protects against all types of UV rays, and as a cream, it is good to protect the skin folds.

Appendix D: Recommended Websites for Patients and Survivors

Here are several recommended websites for cancer patients and survivors. Although it is by no means a complete list of all helpful websites, it is a good place to start.

American Academy of Dermatology	www.aad.org/for-the-public/home
American Cancer Society	www.cancer.org
American College of Radiology	www.radiologyinfo.org
American Society of Clinical Oncology patient site	www.cancer.net
BreastCancer.org	www.breastcancer.org
Cancer Patient Education Network	www.cancerpatienteducation.org
Cancer*Care*	www.cancercare.org
Caring4Cancer	www.caring4cancer.com
Chemocare	www.chemocare.com
Dr. Scholl's	www.drscholls.com
Lindi Skin	www.lindiskin.com
Look Good...Feel Better	www.lookgoodfeelbetter.org
Mayo Clinic	www.mayoclinic.com
Memorial Sloan-Kettering Cancer Center	www.mskcc.org
Multinational Association of Supportive Care in Cancer	www.mascc.org

National Cancer Institute	www.cancer.gov
National Coalition for Cancer Survivorship	www.canceradvocacy.org
National Comprehensive Cancer Network patient site	www.nccn.com
Patient Resource Cancer Guide	www.patientresource.com

Appendix E:
Selected Bibliography

Agha, Rania, et al. "Dermatologic Challenges in Cancer Patients and Survivors." *Oncology (Williston Park)* 21.2 (2007): 1462–72.

Aistars, Juli. "The Validity of Skin Care Protocols Followed by Women with Breast Cancer Receiving External Radiation." *Clinical Journal of Oncology Nursing* 10.4 (2006): 487–92.

Baker, B.W., et al. "Busulphan/Cyclophosphamide Conditioning for Bone Marrow Transplantation May Lead to Failure of Hair Regrowth." *Bone Marrow Transplantation* 7.1 (1991): 43–7.

Baker, C.G. "Moisturization: New Methods to Support Time Proven Ingredients." *Cosmetics and Toiletries* 102.4 (1987): 99–102.

Balagula, Yevgeniy, Mario E. Lacouture, and Jonathan A. Cotliar. "Dermatologic Toxicities of Targeted Anticancer Therapies." *Journal of Supportive Oncology* 8.4 (2010): 149–61.

Balagula, Yevgeniy, et al. "Clinical Presentation and Management of Dermatological Toxicities of Epidermal Growth Factor Receptor Inhibitors." *International Journal of Dermatology* 50.2 (2011): 129–46.

Bergstrom, Kendra G. "Sunscreen Update: The Controversies, What's Safe, What's Next." *Journal of Drugs in Dermatology* 9.11 (2010): 1451–4.

Chen et al. "Grading Dermatologic Adverse Events to Cancer Therapies: The Common Terminology Criteria for Adverse Events (CTCAE), Version 4.0." *Journal of the American Academy of Dermatology* (in press).

Christodoulou, Christos, et al. "Scalp Metastases and Scalp Cooling for Chemotherapy-Induced Alopecia Prevention." *Annals of Oncology* 17.2 (2006): 350.

De Groot, A.C., J.W. Weyland, and J.P. Nater. *Unwanted Effects of Cosmetics and Drugs Used in Dermatology.* Amsterdam: Elsevier, 1994. 498–500.

Draelos, Zoe Diana, and Robert Louis Rietschel. "Hypoallergenicity and the Dermatologist's Perception." *Journal of the American Academy of Dermatology* 35.2 (1996): 248–51.

Dranitsaris, George, et al. "Development and Validation of a Prediction Index for Hand-Foot Skin Reaction in Cancer Patients Receiving Sorafenib." *Annals of Oncology* (2012). Epub ahead of print.

Duvic, Madeleine, et al. "A Randomized Trial of Minoxidil in Chemotherapy-Induced Alopecia." *Journal of the American Academy of Dermatology* 35.1 (1996): 74–8.

Ferrara, James L.M., et al. "Graft-versus-Host Disease." *Lancet* 373.9674 (2009): 1550–61.

Franz, Michael G., David L. Steed, Martin C. Robson. "Optimizing Healing of the Acute Wound by Minimizing Complications." *Current Problems in Surgery* 44.11 (2007): 691–763.

Freedman, Gary M., et al. "Breast Intensity-Modulated Radiation Therapy Reduces Time Spent with Acute Dermatitis for Women of All Breast Sizes during Radiation." *International Journal of Radiation Oncology • Biology • Physics* 74.3 (2009): 689–94.

García-Donoso, Carmen, et al. "Eosinophilic, Polymorphic and Pruritic Eruption Associated with Radiotherapy (EPPER) in Two Patients with Breast Tumour." *Journal of the European Academy of Dermatology and Venereology* 21.8 (2007): 1102–4.

Gilbar, Peter, Alice Hain, and Veta-Marie Peereboom. "Nail Toxicity Induced by Cancer Chemotherapy." *Journal of Oncology Pharmacy Practice* 15.3 (2009): 143–55.

Giralt, Sergio, and Michael R. Bishop. "Principles and Overview of Allogeneic Hematopoietic Stem Cell Transplantation." *Cancer Treatment and Research* 144 (2009): 1–21.

Gonzaga, Evelyn R. "Role of UV Light in Photodamage, Skin Aging, and Skin Cancer: Importance of Photoprotection." *American Journal of Clinical Dermatology* 10. (2009): 19–24.

Graham, Peter H., and J.L. Graham. "Use of Deodorants during Adjuvant Breast Radiotherapy: A Survey of Compliance with Standard Advice, Impact on Patients and a Literature Review on Safety." *Journal of Medical Imaging and Radiation Oncology* 53.6 (2009): 569–73.

Green, Adèle C., et al. "Reduced Melanoma After Regular Sunscreen Use: Randomized Trial Follow-Up." *Journal of Clinical Oncology* 29.3 (2011): 257–63. Epub 2010 Dec 6.

Grevelman, E.G., W.P. Breed. "Prevention of Chemotherapy-Induced Hair Loss by Scalp Cooling." *Annals of Oncology* 16.3 (2005): 352–58.

Hackbarth, Mark, et al. "Chemotherapy-Induced Dermatological Toxicity: Frequencies and Impact on Quality of Life in Women's Cancers: Results of a Prospective Study." *Supportive Care in Cancer* 16.3 (2008): 267–73.

Haley, Ann Cameron, et al. Skin Care Management in Cancer Patients: An Evaluation of Quality of Life and Tolerability. *Supportive Care in Cancer* 19.4 (2011): 545–54.

Hanahan, Douglas, and Robert A. Weinberg. "The Hallmarks of Cancer." *Cell* 100.1 (2000): 57–70.

Heidary, Noushin, Haley Naik, and Susan Burgin. "Chemotherapeutic Agents and the Skin: An Update." *Journal of the American Academy of Dermatology* 58.4 (2008): 545–70.

Hendrichova, I., et al. "Pressure Ulcers in Cancer Palliative Care Patients." *Palliative Medicine* 24.7 (2010): 669–73.

Hesketh, Paul J., et al. "Chemotherapy-induced Alopecia: Psychosocial Impact and Therapeutic Approaches." *Supportive Care in Cancer* 12.8 (2004): 543–9.

Hilton, Shona, et al. "Have Men Been Overlooked? A Comparison of Young Men and Women's Experiences of Chemotherapy-Induced Alopecia." *Psycho-Oncology* 17.6 (2008): 577–83.

Ignatov, A., et al. "An 11-Year Retrospective Study of Totally Implanted Central Venous Access Ports: Complications and Patient Satisfaction." *European Journal of Surgical Oncology* 35.3 (2009): 241–6.

Kassab, Sosie, et al. "Homeopathic Medicines for Adverse Effects of Cancer Treatments." *Cochrane Database of Systematic Reviews* 2 (2009): CD004845.

Kiliç, Arzu, Ülker Gül, and Seçil Soylu. "Skin Findings in Internal Malignant Diseases." *International Journal of Dermatology* 46.10 (2007): 1055–60.

Kinahan, Karen E., et al. "Scarring, Disfigurement and Quality of Life in Long-Term Survivors of Childhood Cancer: A Report from the Childhood Cancer Survivor Study." *Journal of Clinical Oncology* (2012). In press.

Kligman, Lorraine H., Chen Hong Duo, and Albert M. Kligman. "Topical Retinoic Acid Enhances the Repair of Ultraviolet Damaged Dermal Connective Tissue." *Connective Tissue Research* 12.2 (1984): 139–50.

Krasin, Matthew J., et al. "Incidence and Correlates of Radiation Dermatitis in Children and Adolescents Receiving Radiation Therapy for the Treatment of Paediatric Sarcomas." *Clinical Oncology* 21.10 (2009): 781–5.

Lacouture, Mario E. "Mechanisms of Cutaneous Toxicities to EGFR Inhibitors." *Nature Reviews Cancer* 6.10 (2006): 803–12.

Lacouture, Mario E., et al. "Analysis of Dermatologic Events in Patients with Cancer Treated with Lapatinib." *Breast Cancer Research and Treatment* 114.3 (2009): 485–93.

Lawenda, Brian D., et al. "Permanent Alopecia After Cranial Irradiation: Dose-Response Relationship." *International Journal of Radiation Oncology • Biology • Physics* 60.3 (2004): 879–87.

Lorusso, Domenica, et al. "Pegylated Liposomal Doxorubicin-Related Palmar-Plantar Eryth-rodysesthesia ('Hand-Foot' Syndrome)." *Annals of Oncology* 18.7 (2007): 1159–64.

Maibach, Howard I., and Patricia G. Engasser. "Dermatitis Due to Cosmetics." *Contact Dermatitis.* Ed. Alexander A. Fisher. 3rd ed. Philadelphia: Lea & Febiger, 1986. 368–93.

Maida, Vincent, et al. "Wounds and Survival in Cancer Patients." *European Journal of Cancer* 45.18 (2009): 3237-44. Epub 2009 May 28.

Morganti, Alessio G., et al. "Radioprotective Effect of Moderate Wine Consumption in Patients with Breast Carcinoma." *International Journal of Radiation Oncology • Biology • Physics* 74.5 (2009):1501–5.

Neben-Wittich, Michelle A., et al. "Comparison of Provider-Assessed and Patient-Reported Outcome Measures of Acute Skin Toxicity during a Phase III Trial of Mometasone Cream Versus Placebo during Breast Radiotherapy: The North Central Cancer Treatment Group (N06C4)." *International Journal of Radiation Oncology • Biology • Physics* 81.2 (2010): 397–402.

Nymann, Peter, Lene Hedelund, and Merete Haedersdal. "Intense Pulsed Light vs Long-Pulsed Dye Laser Treatment of Telangiectasia After Radiotherapy for Breast Cancer: A Randomized Split-Lesion Trial of Two Different Treatments." *British Journal of Dermatology* 160.6 (2009): 1237–41.

Ogawa, Rei, et al. "Is Radiation Therapy for Keloids Acceptable: The Risk of Radiation-Induced Carcinogenesis." *Plastic and Reconstructive Surgery* 124.4 (2009): 1196–1201.

Paczesny, Sophie, et al. "New Perspectives on the Biology of Acute GVHD." *Bone Marrow Transplantation* 45.1 (2010): 1–11.

Pardo Masferrer, José, et al. "Prophylaxis with a Cream Containing Urea Reduces the Incidence and Severity of Radio-Induced Dermatitis." *Clinical and Translational Oncology* 12.1 (2010): 43–8.

Pasquini, Marcelo C., and Zhiwei Wang. "Current Use and Outcome of Hematopoietic Stem Cell Transplantation." *CIBMTR Summary Slides.* 2010. <http://www.cibmtr.org/ReferenceCenter/SlidesReports/SummarySlides/index.html>.

Patel, Tejesh, and Gil Yosipovitch. "Therapy of Pruritus." *Expert Opinion on Pharmacotherapy* 11.10 (2010): 1673–82.

Perkins, Joanna L., et al. "Nonmelanoma Skin Cancer in Survivors of Childhood and Adolescent Cancer: A Report from the Childhood Cancer Survivor Study." *Journal of Clinical Oncology* 23.16 (2005): 3733–41.

Piraccini, Bianca Maria, et al. "Drug-Induced Nail Diseases." *Dermatologic Clinics* 24.3 (2006): 387–91.

Proksch, Ehrhardt. "The Role of Emollients in the Management of Diseases with Chronic Dry Skin." *Skin Pharmacology and Physiology* 21 (2008): 75–80.

Ramos-Casals, Manuel, et al. "Treatment of Primary Sjögren Syndrome: A Systematic Review." *Journal of the American Medical Association* 304.4 (2010): 452–60.

Ryan, Julie L., et al. "Post-Treatment Skin Reactions Reported by Cancer Patients Differ by Race, Not by Treatment or Expectations." *British Journal of Cancer* 97 (2007): 14–21.

Salvo, N., et al. "Prophylaxis and Management of Acute Radiation-Induced Skin Reactions: A Systematic Review of the Literature." *Current Oncology* 17.4 (2010): 94–112.

Samaras, Panagiotis, et al. "Infectious Port Complications Are More Frequent in Younger Patients with Hematologic Malignancies Than in Solid Tumor Patients." *Oncology* 74 (2008): 237–44.

Şanli, Hatice, et al. "Clinical Manifestations of Cutaneous Graft-versus-Host Disease After Allogeneic Haematopoietic Cell Transplantation: Long-Term Follow-Up Results in a Single Turkish Centre." *Acta Dermato Venereologica* 84 (2004): 296–301.

Sasse, André Deeke, et al. "Amifostine Reduces Side Effects and Improves Complete Response Rate during Radiotherapy: Results of a Meta-Analysis." *International Journal of Radiation Oncology • Biology • Physics* 64 (2006): 784–91.

Scheinfeld, Noah, Maurice J. Dahdah, and Richard Scher. "Vitamins and Minerals: Their Role in Nail Health and Disease." *Journal of Drugs in Dermatology* 6.8 (2007): 782–7.

Scotté, Florian, et al. "Multicenter Study of a Frozen Glove to Prevent Docetaxel-Induced Onycholysis and Cutaneous Toxicity of the Hand." *Journal of Clinical Oncology* 23 (2005): 4424–9.

Sherber, N.S., et al. "Efficacy and Safety Study of Tazarotene Cream 0.1% for the Treatment of Brittle Nail Syndrome." *Cutis* 87 (2011): 96–103.

Sidle, Douglas M., and Haena Kim. "Keloids: Prevention and Management." *Facial Plastic Surgery Clinics of North America* 19.3 (2011): 505–15.

Sonis, Steven T. "Oral Mucositis." *Anti-cancer Drugs* 22.7 (2011): 607–12.

Ständer, Sonja, et al. "Targeting the Neurokinin Receptor 1 with Aprepitant: A Novel Antipruritic Strategy." *PLoS One* 5.6 (2010): e10968.

Szymanski, Konrad M., et al. "External Stoma and Peristomal Complications Following Radical Cystectomy and Ileal Conduit Diversion: A Systematic Review." *Ostomy Wound Management* 56.1 (2010): 28–35.

Tallon, Ben, Elizabeth Blanchard, and Lynne J. Goldberg. "Permanent Chemotherapy-Induced Alopecia: Case Report and Review of the Literature." *Journal of the American Academy of Dermatology* 63 (2010): 333–6.

Tejwani, Ajay, et al. "Increased Risk of High-Grade Dermatologic Toxicities with Radiation plus Epidermal Growth Factor Receptor Inhibitor Therapy." *Cancer* 115 (2009): 1286–99.

Théberge, Valérie, François Harel, and Anne Dagnault. "Use of Axillary Deodorant and Effect on Acute Skin Toxicity during Radiotherapy for Breast Cancer: A Prospective Randomized Noninferiority Trial." *International Journal of Radiation Oncology • Biology • Physics* 75.4 (2009): 1048–52.

Thiers, Bruce H., Rachel E. Sahn, and Jeffrey E. Callen. "Cutaneous Manifestations of Internal Malignancy." *CA: A Cancer Journal for Clinicians* 59.2 (2009): 73–98.

Ulrik, A.F., and S. Matzen. "Studies of Injection Ports of Permanent Expandable Breast Implants." *Journal of Plastic, Reconstructive, and Aesthetic Surgery* 63 (2010): 327–31.

Vowels M., et al. "Factors Affecting Hair Regrowth After Bone Marrow Transplantation." *Bone Marrow Transplantation* 12 (1993): 347–50.

Wallace, W.H.B., and D.M. Green, eds. *Late Effects of Childhood Cancer.* London: Arnold Publishers, 2004.

Wang, Jie, Ze Lu, and Jessie L.-S. Au. "Protection Against Chemotherapy-Induced Alopecia." *Pharmaceutical Research* 23 (2006): 2505–14.

Wang, Steven Q., Yevgeniy Balagula, and Uli Osterwalder. "Photoprotection: A Review of the Current and Future Technologies." *Dermatologic Therapy* 23.1 (2010): 31–47.

Wells, F.V., and Irvin I. Lubowe. *Cosmetics and the Skin.* New York: Reinhold Publishing Corporation, 1964. 141–9.

Zawacki, Walter J., et al. "Wound Dehiscence or Failure to Heal Following Venous Access Port Placement in Patients Receiving Bevacizumab Therapy." *Journal of Vascular and Interventional Radiology* 20 (2009): 624–27.

Index

A

B

C

melanoma 4–5, 50, 72, 84, 114, 161, 225, 242
multiple myeloma 9, 166–168, 184
myelodysplastic syndrome 73, 167–168, 184
neuroendocrine cancer 6, 104
non-Hodgkin lymphoma 55, 168, 242
ovarian cancer 4–6, 48, 84, 114, 145, 154, 210
pancreatic cancer 6, 8, 72, 146
prostate cancer 46, 72, 104, 124–125, 145, 205, 228
skin cancer 5, 8, 138, 150, 181, 185–186, 189, 198, 200, 225–226, 236, 241, 243, 245
squamous cell carcinoma 5
stomach cancer 6–8, 72, 106, 128
testicular cancer 6, 242
thyroid cancer 6, 8, 9
uterine cancer 6, 145
Capecitabine 16, 29, 44, 48, 74–75, 89, 105, 188, 224, 229, 231
Captopril 12
Carboplatin 27, 105, 111, 138, 225, 229
Carmustine 105, 224
Cellulitis 38, 53, 148
Cervical cancer. *See* Cancer
Cetirizine 21, 38, 79, 80, 82, 178
Cetuximab 14–15, 24, 27, 29–30, 32, 35, 44, 51, 66–67, 73–75, 88–89, 92, 96, 98–99, 105, 107, 109–111, 128, 188, 198, 224, 227, 231
Childhood cancer. *See* Cancer
Chlorambucil 75, 105, 111, 138, 188
Chronic myelogenous leukemia. *See* Cancer
Ciprofloxacin 24, 87, 96–97, 160, 188
Cisplatin 20, 27, 105, 111, 138
Cladribine 27, 37, 75
Clindamycin 23, 34
Clobetasol 19, 21, 35, 42, 48, 62, 84, 159–160, 240
Codeine 12, 42, 48, 75–76, 78, 132, 149
Cold caps 112–114
Colon cancer. *See* Cancer
Colorectal cancer. *See* Cancer
Concealer 211–212, 216
Coping
  hair loss 101–102, 111–112
  improving self-image 204–205
Corticosteroids 7, 12, 14, 18–21, 24, 28, 30, 32, 34–36, 38–40, 42, 46, 48, 67, 69–70, 76–77, 79, 81–84, 107, 126, 128–130, 132, 134, 137, 140, 147–148, 150–153, 159–160, 164, 173, 175, 178, 180, 189, 205–207, 215, 227, 232, 236, 239–240, 242–243
Cosmeceuticals 206, 214

Cosmetics 206–221
  acne and 204–205
  application 209–214
  choice 207–208, 212–213
  infections and 208
  natural ingredients 218–219
  safety 203–204, 218–221
  self-image 204–205
  what to avoid 210–211
Cyclophosphamide 27–30, 32, 34, 44, 74–75, 89, 105, 111, 138, 174, 224–225, 229
Cyclosporine 174
Cytarabine 27, 29, 37, 48, 75, 104–105, 168, 173–174

D

Dacarbazine 37, 89, 105, 188, 229
Dactinomycin 104
Dalteparin 75
Darbepoetin alfa 75
Dasatinib 29, 37, 39, 44, 74–75, 105, 110, 188, 224
Daunorubicin 37, 42, 75, 89, 105, 229, 242
Deferasirox 16
Dehydration 58
Dexamethasone 12, 19, 35–36, 38, 40, 48, 82–83, 132, 175, 178, 180, 239, 242
Diltiazem 44
Diphenhydramine 21, 38, 66, 74, 79–81, 132, 137, 173, 178, 189
Docetaxel 20, 27–30, 32, 34, 39, 44, 66, 74–75, 85, 88–89, 96, 98–99, 102, 105, 116, 134, 188, 224–225, 227, 229, 231
Doxepin 21–22, 74, 81–83, 178
Doxorubicin 29, 35–37, 41–42, 44, 48, 74–75, 89, 104–105, 113, 134, 164, 224, 229, 231, 242
Doxycycline 24, 188
Dry eyes 66–67
Dry lips 215
Dry mouth 67–69, 135–136, 236
  treatment 68
Dry skin
  causes 54–56
  cracks 60
  grading severity 53–54
  management 61–65, 128
  prevention and treatment 55–65

E

Eczema 22, 53, 55
Eltrombopag 16
Endometrial cancer. *See* Cancer
Enoxaparin 12, 75

About the Author

Mario E. Lacouture, MD

Dr. Lacouture is a board-certified dermatologist with a special interest in dermatologic conditions that result from cancer treatments. His clinical focus is the recognition and management of the side effects and conditions of the skin, hair, and nails that may arise in cancer patients and survivors as a consequence of chemotherapy, radiation, or transplantation. His research focuses on exploring new skin treatments that do not interfere with the effectiveness of anticancer drugs. Dr. Lacouture received his MD degree from Javeriana University in Colombia. He completed residencies at Cleveland Clinic Foundation and the University of Chicago Hospital, and a fellowship at Brigham and Women's Hospital. Prior to his current position as an Associate Member at Memorial Sloan-Kettering Cancer Center, he was on the attending staff at Northwestern University's Feinberg School of Medicine, where he founded the SERIES clinic. Dr. Lacouture has received numerous grants and awards, has published more than 90 scientific papers, and is listed as one of "America's Best Doctors." He lives in New York City.

Cornelia Dean

Ms. Dean is a science writer and former science editor of *The New York Times,* where she writes about science policy, environmental issues, and related topics. She offers regular seminars at Harvard University on the public's understanding of science. From January 1997 until June 2003, as science editor of *The Times,* she was responsible for coverage of science, health, and medical news in the daily paper and in the weekly Science Times section. In 2003, she was a Shorenstein Fellow at the Kennedy School of Government at Harvard. Her first book, *Against the Tide: The Battle for America's Beaches,* was published in 1999 by Columbia University Press and was a New York Times Notable Book of the Year. Her guide for scientists on the communication of science, *Am I Making Myself Clear?,* was published in 2009 by Harvard University Press. She is at work on a book about the misuse of scientific information in American public life.

Steven T. Rosen, MD, FACP

Dr. Rosen is the Genevieve E. Teuton Professor of Medicine and Director of the Robert H. Lurie Comprehensive Cancer Center of Northwestern University. Following his graduation with distinction from Northwestern University Medical School's Honors Program, Dr. Rosen completed his residency in Internal Medicine at Northwestern and a fellowship in Medical Oncology at the National Cancer Institute (NCI). Dr. Rosen's laboratory investigations focus on experimental therapeutics and hematologic malignancies. He has received numerous awards, grants, and contracts and has published more than 300 scientific papers. Dr. Rosen serves on the advisory boards of several NCI-designated Cancer Centers, the Leukemia and Lymphoma Society of America, the Multiple Myeloma Research Foundation, the Cure for Lymphoma Foundation, and the Wendy Will Cancer Research Foundation. Dr. Rosen also is listed as one of "Chicago's Top Doctors" and "America's Top Doctors."

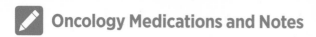

Oncology Medications and Notes

Use this page to create a record of the medications prescribed by your oncologist, including chemotherapies, targeted therapies, antibiotics, and corticosteroids. Bring this book to your doctor's appointment so that you may share the most accurate information possible with your caregivers.

Medication Name, Generic (Trade, if available): _____
Number of cycles or weeks: _____ Last received: _____
Purpose: _____
Comments: _____

Medication Name, Generic (Trade, if available): _____
Number of cycles or weeks: _____ Last received: _____
Purpose: _____
Comments: _____

Medication Name, Generic (Trade, if available): _____
Number of cycles or weeks: _____ Last received: _____
Purpose: _____
Comments: _____

Medication Name, Generic (Trade, if available): _____
Number of cycles or weeks: _____ Last received: _____
Purpose: _____
Comments: _____

Medication Name, Generic (Trade, if available): _____
Number of cycles or weeks: _____ Last received: _____
Purpose: _____
Comments: _____

Medication Name, Generic (Trade, if available): _____
Number of cycles or weeks: _____ Last received: _____
Purpose: _____
Comments: _____

Medication Name, Generic (Trade, if available): _____
Number of cycles or weeks: _____ Last received: _____
Purpose: _____
Comments: _____